Protecting the
World's Children

Protecting the World's Children
Immunisation policies and practices

Edited by

Sidsel Roalkvam

Desmond McNeill

Stuart Blume

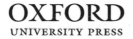

OXFORD
UNIVERSITY PRESS

OXFORD
UNIVERSITY PRESS

Great Clarendon Street, Oxford, OX2 6DP,
United Kingdom

Oxford University Press is a department of the University of Oxford.
It furthers the University's objective of excellence in research, scholarship,
and education by publishing worldwide. Oxford is a registered trade mark of
Oxford University Press in the UK and in certain other countries

First Edition published in 2013

Impression: 1

Published in the United States of America by Oxford University Press
198 Madison Avenue, New York, NY 10016, United States of America

British Library Cataloguing in Publication Data

Data available

Library of Congress Control Number: 2013937328

ISBN 978–0–19–966644–7

Printed in Great Britain by
CPI Group (UK) Ltd, Croydon, CR0 4YY

Oxford University Press makes no representation, express or implied, that the
drug dosages in this book are correct. Readers must therefore always check
the product information and clinical procedures with the most up-to-date
published product information and data sheets provided by the manufacturers
and the most recent codes of conduct and safety regulations. The authors and
the publishers do not accept responsibility or legal liability for any errors in the
text or for the misuse or misapplication of material in this work. Except where
otherwise stated, drug dosages and recommendations are for the non-pregnant
adult who is not breast-feeding

Links to third party websites are provided by Oxford in good faith and
for information only. Oxford disclaims any responsibility for the materials
contained in any third party website referenced in this work.

Preface

We embarked on this study of immunisation policies and practices in 2008. Our intention was to use immunisation as a lens for viewing the dilemmas of development in the 21st century. Vaccines and immunisation exemplify many of the incongruities of today's globalising world: global but also local, high technology brought to intimate and personal spheres, transnational industry producing what are said to be public goods, appeals made both to individual choice and to collective responsibility.

How are vaccines used in practice? How could they best be deployed in the interests of the health and development of children in poor countries? These were the questions on which the multidisciplinary research project SUM Medic, based at the Centre for Development and the Environment at the University of Oslo, was to focus. Whilst immunisation is often referred to as a simple and cost-effective technique of child protection, its practice is embedded in socially, politically, and technically complex structures. The predominant view from a public health perspective is that if supply chains function properly, if populations are ensured access, then high immunisation coverage will follow. Yet this is too simple. Today there are large variations in immunisation coverage, both between countries and between regions of a single country. Similarly, the adoption of new and improved vaccines, which varies from country to country, does not follow conventional measures of development, such as per capita income. Some low-income countries, such as Malawi, have higher average immunisation coverage than, for example, India. Similarly, Rwanda adopts new vaccines at the same rate as many middle-income countries. How can these differences, between nations and between communities, be understood? We wanted to open up and explore the decision-making processes that take place as individuals, communities, and nations make choices about the vaccines accessible to them.

Both the research and this book have been a team effort in every sense of the term. The original research on which the book draws involved researchers from India, Malawi, the Netherlands, Norway, and the USA. Our work has also been highly interdisciplinary, with contributions from public health, social anthropology, economics, political science and international relations, and political economy. Trying to integrate distinctive disciplinary perspectives, as each of the chapters of this book does, has been challenging. It has forced each of us to think critically about the assumptions and the methods that our disciplines tend to take for granted. We have been reminded of the sense of curiosity that brought us into intellectual work in the first place, and of the constraints that disciplinary training and perspectives can produce.

The form of this book is rather unusual. Although an edited volume, its preparation has been very different from the way most edited volumes come about. The reader will certainly be struck by the fact that where one chapter refers to something in another, we use formulations like 'as we noted earlier', even though the chapters have different authors. The contributors have been working on this study over a number of years. Regular workshops have taken place at which progress and findings have been discussed with a wide range of additional experts in international health. The structure of the book and the focus of individual chapters have been discussed and developed over time. Each of us has profited from the intellectual confrontations involved in working and writing with colleagues from other backgrounds. Nevertheless some differences in interpretation remain. The 'we' of the final chapter of the book, drawing things together, refers to the authors of that chapter. We would not wish to commit all contributors to the interpretations we give there.

As a team we would like to express our appreciation to the research students who made an invaluable contribution to our empirical work: Kristin Alfsen, Ellen Eie, Lotte Danielsen, Dagrun Kyte Gjøstein, John Holte, Synnøve Knivestøen, and Mette Ommundsen. They conducted great fieldwork and developed their findings in excellent theses. In India, similarly, we thank MA students Sumita Sarma and Shefali Hasija for their excellent contributions. In Malawi and India our research was ably supported by local assistants Anita and Manju, and local advisor Dr Soubhagya Padhy. We thank them for their substantial contributions to the studies.

Our research, however, would not have been possible if not for the many people within Malawi, India, and the global community who made time to meet and share their views and experiences with us. We wish to extend our thanks to governmental officials in the Malawi government, in particular the Ministry of Health, to officials in UN agencies, foundations, CHAM, and NGO representatives. In India we are grateful to representatives from the Indian Government (Ministry of Biotechnology and the Ministry of Health and Family Welfare), public health activists, representatives of WHO India, the leadership of the GAVI-funded Hib Initiative, and representatives of GAVI and the NGO PATH, in both Geneva and New Delhi. Not least we are indebted to the many local communities in both Malawi and India that have provided not only information but homes, comfort, and support for researchers and fieldworkers.

Our research has been generously funded over 4 years (2008–2012) by the Research Council of Norway under the GLOBVAC programme. The additional technical and enthusiastic support from GLOBVAC coordinator Kårstein Måseide has been invaluable. We also wish to extend thanks to the institutional support given by the Sociology Department at the Delhi School of Economics and the Public Health Foundation in India, and the Reach Trust in Malawi for providing our intellectual home away from home. Finally, our appreciation goes to our colleagues at the Centre for Development and the Environment (SUM) at the University of Oslo for providing such a good home and anchorage for this multisited and multipartnership project. We express our gratitude to our Director Kristi Anne Stølen and administrative staff Gitte Egenberg, Hans Jørgen Christiansen, Kristoffer Ring, and Knut Kjæreng for tirelessly providing us with administrative support.

Sidsel Roalkvam
Oslo, May 2013

Contents

Abbreviations

AFP	acute flaccid paralysis
AMP	Agence de Médicine Préventive
ANM	auxiliary nurse midwife
ASHA	accredited social health activist
AWW	Angan Wadi worker
BCG	Bacillus Calmette–Guérin
BCMO	block chief medical officer
BMGF	Bill and Melinda Gates Foundation
CDC	Centers for Disease Control and Prevention
CHAI	Clinton Health Access Initiative
CHAM	Christian Medical Association of Malawi
CHC	community health centres
CSSM	Child Survival and Safe Motherhood Programme
CVI	Children's Vaccine Initiative
CVP	Children's Vaccine Programme
DALY	disability-adjusted life year
DANIDA	Danish International Development Agency
DfID	Department for International Development (UK)
DHS	Demographic and Health Survey
DNA	deoxyribonucleic acid
DPTP	diphtheria, pertussis, tetanus, and polio vaccine
DRDO	Defence Research and Development Organization
DTP	(also DPT) diphtheria, tetanus, and pertussis vaccine
EHP	essential health package
EPI	expanded programme of immunization
FDA	Food and Drug Administration
GAVI	Global Alliance for Vaccines and Immunisation
GOBI	growth monitoring, oral rehydration therapy, breast feeding, and immunisation
GPPP	global public–private partnerships
GSK	GlaxoSmithKline
H1N1	new influenza, 'Mexican flu' or 'swine flu'
HEU	health education unit
Hib	haemophilus influenzae type b
HIV AIDS	human immunodeficiency virus infection/acquired immunodeficiency syndrome
HMIS	health management information system
HPV	human papilloma virus
HSA	health surveillance assistant
HSS	health systems strengthening
IAVI	International AIDS Vaccine Initiative
ICC	Interagency Coordination Committee
ICMR	Indian Council of Medical Research
IFPMA	International Federation of Pharmaceutical Manufacturers and Associations
IHR	International Health Regulations
IUD	intrauterine device
JICA	Japanese International Cooperation Agency
KfW	Kreditanstalt für Wiederaufbau (The German Development Bank)
LLR	Lanzhou lamb rotavirus
MCHN	mother–child health and nutrition
MDG	millennium development goal
MDHS	Malawi Demographic and Health Survey

MICS	multiple indicator cluster surveys	SAGE	Strategic Advisory Group of Experts on Immunisation
MMR	measles, mumps, and rubella vaccine	SARS	severe acute respiratory syndrome
MO	medical officer	SC	scheduled castes
MoH	Ministry of Health	ST	scheduled tribes
MoHFW	Ministry of Health and Family Welfare	SWAp	sector-wide approach
		TB	tuberculosis
MSF	Médecins Sans Frontières (Doctors without Borders)	TBA	traditional birth attendants
		TT	tetanus toxoid
MVI	Malaria Vaccine Initiative	UCI	Universal Childhood Immunization
NFHS	National Family Health Survey		
NGO	non-governmental organisation	UIP	Universal Immunization Programme
NIAID	National Institute of Allergy and Infectious Diseases		
		UN	United Nations
NIDs	national immunisation days	UNAIDS	United Nations Programme on HIV/AIDS
Norad	Norwegian Agency for Development Cooperation		
		UNDP	United Nations Development Programme
NRHM	National Rural Health Mission		
NTAGI	National Technical Advisory Group on Immunization	UNFPA	United Nations Fund for Population Activities
NUVI	New and Under-utilized Vaccines Introduction	UNHCR	United Nations High Commissioner for Refugees
OECD	Organisation for Economic Co-operation and Development	UNICEF	United Nations Children's Fund
OPV	oral polio vaccine	UPI	Universal Programme on Immunization
ORT	oral rehydation therapy		
PAHO	Pan American Health Organisation	USAID	United States Agency for International Development
PHC	primary health centre	VAERS	vaccine-adverse event reporting system
PIE	post-introduction evaluation		
PPP	public–private partnership	VPD	vaccine-preventable diseases
RCH	Reproductive and Child Health Programme	WG	Working Group
		WHA	World Health Assembly
R0	reproductive rate	WHO	World Health Organization

Contributors

Steinar Andresen
Research Professor
Fridtjof Nansen Institute
Polhøgda, Norway

Stuart Blume
Emeritus Professor
Department of Sociology
and Anthropology
University of Amsterdam,
the Netherlands

Rune Flikke
Associate Professor
Department of Social Anthropology
University of Oslo, Norway

Jagrati Jani
Postdoctoral Fellow
Institute of Health and Society
Faculty of Medicine
University of Oslo, Norway

Judith Justice
Associate Professor Medical
Anthropology and of Health Policy
School of Medicine
University of California,
San Francisco (UCSF), USA

Desmond McNeill
Professor
Centre for Development
and the Environment
University of Oslo, Norway

Arima Mishra
Faculty
Institute of Public Health
Bangalore, India

Cecilie Nordfeldt
Research Fellow
Department of Social Anthropology
University of Oslo, Norway

Lot Nyirenda
Research Fellow
Centre for Development
and the Environment
University of Oslo, Norway

Sidsel Roalkvam
Associate Professor
Centre for Development
and the Environment
University of Oslo, Norway

Kristin Ingstad Sandberg
Postdoctoral Fellow
Centre for Development
and the Environment
University of Oslo, Norway

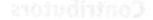

Chapter 1

Saving children's lives: perspectives on immunisation

Stuart Blume, Jagrati Jani,
and Sidsel Roalkvam

Introduction

Vaccines have been crucial tools in the public health armamentarium for decades, and immunisation has long been seen as one of the most effective (and cost-effective) ways of saving children's lives. Because the number of infectious diseases against which a vaccine exists has grown, immunisation schedules have become increasingly complex. For example, in the early 1950s children in the USA were offered four antigens combined in two vaccines: one against smallpox, and one compound DPT (diphtheria, pertussis, and tetanus) vaccine. By the late 1980s, smallpox vaccination had been discontinued and American children were given eight antigens in four vaccines by the time they entered school: DPT, oral polio, MMR (measles, mumps, and rubella), and Hib (haemophilus influenzae type b). The trend continues, and many countries now recommend HPV vaccine (against cervical cancer) for girls in their early teens. Developing countries are urged to speed up the introduction of new vaccines, including those against Hib, hepatitis B, and rotavirus.

Although reliance on vaccines is by no means new to public health, it seems today that their role is becoming ever more central. Vast sums of money are invested in the search for new vaccines against diseases regarded as potentially 'vaccine preventable'. For example, over the past few years nearly US$1 billion has been invested annually in the search for a vaccine against HIV AIDS. When, in 2009, a new influenza virus (H1N1) was identified, there were fears that it would wreak havoc comparable with the Spanish flu of 1918. In June 2009 the World Health Organization (WHO) declared a pandemic, and a dramatic race to produce and distribute a vaccine began immediately. In January 2010 Bill Gates, speaking at the Davos World Economic Forum, called for a 'decade of vaccines', and pledged US$10 billion in support of it. By the end of 2010, the leaders of WHO, the United Nations Children's Fund (UNICEF), and the

American National Institute of Allergy and Infectious Diseases (NIAID, part of the National Institutes of Health) had joined with the Bill and Melinda Gates Foundation (BMGF) in preparations for a Global Vaccines Action Plan. Vaccines are also big business. The global vaccine market is expected to reach US$34 billion in sales in the course of 2012, with a growth rate of 14% forecast for the next 5 years (Center for Vaccine Ethics and Policy 2011).

The contribution that vaccines make to improvements in public health is not determined by their immunological properties alone. It depends also on how they are administered: on the effective organisation of immunisation programmes. In the case of some diseases (including smallpox, diphtheria, measles, and polio) substantial benefits accrue when a very high proportion of the eligible population (80 or 90%) are immunised: the exact percentage depends on the virulence of the pathogen and the efficacy of the vaccine. Thanks to this 'herd (or community) immunity' effect, people who have not been immunised are also protected when coverage exceeds this threshold value. In other words, whatever the efficacy of a vaccine in protecting the individual child, the collective benefit depends on the share of the population that has been vaccinated.

Despite past successes immunisation programmes still function far from perfectly, and in 2005 WHO and UNICEF jointly announced a new 'global strategy'. It would have four elements:

> The global strategy proposes to sustain immunization to those who are currently reached, extend immunization to those who are currently unreached and to age groups beyond infancy, introduce new vaccines and technologies and link immunization to other health interventions as well as to the development of the overall health system. It places immunization firmly within the context of sector-wide approaches to health, highlighting the way immunization can both benefit from and contribute to health-system development and the alleviation of system-wide barriers. (WHO/UNICEF 2005, p. 24)

In this book we too will be concerned with the question of how vaccines, as powerful tools of public health, can best be deployed, and with the programmes through which they are provided and the relationships of those programmes to other forms of healthcare provision. A global perspective, however, such as that underlying the WHO/UNICEF strategy, will not be taken for granted in this book. Indeed, one of our objectives will be to show that what may appear to be an effective and successful programme from a global perspective may be viewed very differently from a national level—and vice versa. The local communities and the families living in them, whose myriad decisions ultimately determine the success or failure of an immunisation programme, provide yet further perspectives which, again, may differ from those of public health officials. Where differences in perspective are substantial, plans may be thwarted, implementation ineffective, and even seeds of conflict sown.

In the literature dealing with the functioning, successes, and failings of current immunisation programmes and initiatives, history is used in a very particular way. References to the past are typically limited to a listing of past achievements: the eradication of smallpox or (substantial and quantifiable) reductions in morbidity and mortality from diphtheria, tetanus, measles or polio. With the exception of smallpox eradication, discussed in more detail below, there is rarely much attention to the organisation of vaccination programmes. Yet here too there is a distinct logic, and the ways in which current initiatives build on earlier ones (the phenomenon known to historians as 'path dependency') are significant. Assumptions underlying new initiatives may unconsciously mirror those of previous ones, their goals formulated with respect to what are perceived as the successes and failures of previous programmes, and the resources and structures available for implementation shaped by what has gone before. The global immunisation strategy set out by WHO and UNICEF in 2005 is linked in innumerable ways to the assumptions underlying, the organisation, and the successes and failures of previous strategies and programmes.

It is beyond the scope of this chapter, or indeed of this book, to provide a comprehensive history of immunisation policies, practices, and programmes. Instead, we have selected a number of key episodes that display something of these historic continuities. Thereafter we will use this historical account to articulate a number of elements that have become fundamental to immunisation policy and thinking today.

Immunisation history

From roughly the middle of the 19th century European states began seriously to concern themselves with the health of their populations. Founding heroes of public health include the German pathologist Rudolf Virchow, who in 1848 was sent by the Prussian government to investigate a typhoid epidemic in the coalmining province of Silesia. Living among the miners for some weeks, Virchow concluded that disease could only be understood in terms of the multiple deprivations (poor housing, poor working conditions, lack of sanitation, and so on) from which the community suffered. His recommendations to the Prussian government, which were not welcomed, emphasised the importance of political, social, and economic reform. The founding heroes also include Edwin Chadwick, the British official whose famous report on the deteriorating living and working conditions of the British poor led to passage of the 1848 Public Health Act. It was from the mid-19th century that social reformers like these, not all of them physicians, convinced European governments of the dangers of insanitary conditions and the epidemics to which they often led. Industrial productivity, social order, the effectiveness of armies, and the self-image of a Christian and god-fearing nation: all were placed in jeopardy by the ravages of epidemic disease. By the beginning of the 20th century, however, the focus in public health began to shift away from social and environmental reform. Much influenced by Koch's bacteriological discoveries, it began to move towards the search for the aetiological agents of diseases through laboratory investigations. Public health laboratories were established in Europe, North America, and many far-flung colonies. The protection of their borders against contamination, of their economic and colonial interests, dictated great power involvement in international health. In the 19th century a series of sanitary conferences had emphasised quarantines and the surveillance of travellers in the attempt to prevent the spread of epidemic diseases (cholera, plague, yellow fever) across national borders. Through these international agreements the great powers sought to protect themselves against contamination. By the 20th century, and reflected in the Rockefeller Foundation and the Pasteur Institute's establishment of networks of public health laboratories in Africa, Asia, and Latin America, the basic paradigm of public health was changing. Both the Pasteur Institute and the Rockefeller Foundation 'were active in medical and biological research, and considered medicine as the cornerstone of progress' (Moulin 2004). Both coordinated programmes for controlling or eliminating disease, and 'developed lobbying techniques for influencing governments'. Indeed the Rockefeller Foundation actively sought to secure the strong administrative structures which, outside the USA, it regarded as essential for the containment of epidemics (Moulin 2004).

This shift in focus, public health rooted in biological research and strong, centralised administrative structures was facilitated by new vaccines (against typhoid, tetanus, diphtheria, and tuberculosis) that from the 1920s were becoming available on a large scale. From the 1950s onwards, the number of vaccines available for preventing infectious diseases in children increased rapidly, mainly as a result of developments in virology. Research by John Enders and his Harvard colleagues in the late 1940s, demonstrating the feasibility of safely culturing polio virus, was a vital breakthrough. Enders' work initiated the development of vaccines against a variety of viral diseases. In the USA the first vaccines against polio, measles, and rubella were licensed in 1955, 1963, and 1970, respectively. Further breakthroughs followed, and the first vaccines developed using recombinant DNA technology, against hepatitis B, were licensed at the end of the 1980s.

There are various possible approaches to writing immunisation history (Blume 2008; Gradmann and Hess 2008). One is in terms of scientific progress:

the scientific and technical achievements and the difficulties overcome that have led to production of more, safer, and more effective vaccines. Recognising that lives are only saved if the vaccines are effectively administered to large numbers of people, another approach to this history focuses on the organisation of immunisation programmes. The great successes that have, justifiably, been attributed to immunisation—smallpox eradication, reduction in morbidity, disability and mortality from diphtheria, measles, polio, and other diseases—had to confront parental or bureaucratic apathy, professional doubts, and in some cases popular resistance. They were not achieved overnight.

The long road to smallpox eradication (1801–1980)

In 1801 Edward Jenner, who a few years earlier had demonstrated a procedure for vaccinating against smallpox, suggested that smallpox eradication ought to be possible (Fenner 1996). He was to be proved right, but it was to take 180 years. In many countries laws were passed making vaccination of infants against smallpox compulsory (in England in 1853, in the Netherlands in 1871, in Germany in 1874, and in France in 1902). Although the laws were differently administered in the different countries, organised opposition emerged in many (Blume 2006). In England, for example, parents who could afford it could have their child vaccinated by a medical practitioner. Those who could not were directed to state-paid vaccinators who functioned under the aegis of the Poor Law Guardians. Not only was the whole Poor Law structure and administration seen as cruelly stigmatising, but Poor Law vaccination officers (civil servants appointed to seek out non-compliers) could and did prosecute parents who failed to comply with the law, especially working-class parents. There was widespread resistance, especially among respectable working-class people who might also have been active in the trade union or cooperative movements. Historian Nadja Durbach has shown how an idea of good citizenship was central to the dispute (Durbach 2000). However, vaccination advocates, and members of the national antivaccination movement that had emerged in England by the 1860s, had different understandings of the concept. For the former group, the citizenship of the working class, symbolised by extension of the right to vote, entailed sharing in an obligation to protect the health of the community. By contrast, for the National Anti-Compulsory Vaccination League, good citizenship did not mean enforcing public health measures; rather, it entailed respecting the bodies of fellow citizens.

As the name of the Anti-Compulsory Vaccination League suggests, much of the resistance was against the compulsory nature of vaccination, rather than vaccination itself. Protestors claimed the right to opt out for reasons of conscience.

In 1889, in response to public pressure, the British government appointed a Royal Commission on Vaccination. It took this Commission 7 years to develop compromise proposals allowing for a right to opt out, although it was only in 1907 that the law was changed accordingly. Gradually, with improvements in health services, these movements declined and smallpox in Europe was brought under control. By the mid-1960s, it had virtually disappeared from the USA and Europe, although it was still present in Latin America, Africa, and above all Asia. The liquid vaccine used in Europe was far less effective in tropical conditions (Fenner 1996). It was only with the development of a more stable freeze-dried vaccine, in the early 1950s, that the idea of a worldwide attack on smallpox began to seem feasible. In 1958 the Soviet delegates to the World Health Assembly (WHA) proposed a global smallpox eradication campaign. They argued that transmission would be halted if 80% of the population was vaccinated. The USSR and other countries supplied freeze-dried vaccine to countries in which small-pox was endemic and the disease was eliminated from many smaller countries— but not from the larger countries of Asia and Africa. Even if it could be achieved, it was becoming clear that 80% coverage would be inadequate. Based on the observation in India that smallpox persisted in some areas despite vaccinations reported to be 80% or more of the population, in 1964 the WHO Expert Committee on Smallpox recommended that the goal should be to vaccinate 100% of the population. In 1966 the 19th WHA approved an Intensified Smallpox Eradication programme, and a special Smallpox Eradication Unit, headed by ex-Centers for Disease Control and Prevention (CDC) smallpox chief DA Henderson, was established in Geneva. At that time, official figures suggested a (fluctuating) figure of some 100,000 new cases of smallpox per annum, of which no less than 30–40% were found in India (Bhattacharya 2004). Real figures are likely to have been very much higher. Implementation of the campaign, and the progress made, differed significantly from one area to another. West and Central African countries, for example, made rapid progress, with material and person-nel support from the USA. Between January 1967 and December 1969, 100 mil-lion people were vaccinated against smallpox in the 20-country region (Foege et al. 1975). In May 1970 the last cases were reported there.

The situation in India (which had started its own pilot eradication schemes much earlier) was different, and the WHO-coordinated programme encoun-tered a multitude of political and administrative problems (Bhattarchya 2004). In India, in 1973, there were still tens of thousands of new cases of smallpox annually. The Indian subcontinent was singled out for concentrated interna-tional attention, and large numbers of foreign (mainly American) physician-epidemiologists flown into the region (Greenough 1995). The strategy then adopted was that everyone in a village in which a case of smallpox had been identified was to be vaccinated, irrespective of prior immune status: the so-called 'ring fence' strategy. Coercion was not uncommon, and force was sometimes employed (Greenough 1995). From the perspective of public health the campaign was an unprecedented success. The last case of smallpox was located (in Somalia) in 1977 and in May 1980 the WHA adopted a resolution declaring that smallpox had been eradicated.

Widely hailed as public health's greatest triumph, the smallpox eradication programme has been highly influential in showing the feasibility of disease eradication as a public health goal, and in attesting to the benefits of globally coordinated public health programmes. It had led to development of the ring fence immunisation strategy and, as we shall show presently, it inspired, and to some extent provided the infrastructure for, the Expanded Programme of Immunization. Yet history can be read in different ways, and a few historians of public health have offered a different interpretation. Paul Greenough, for example, has argued that however justifiable coercive and aggressive values might have been in the context of an eradication campaign, they are inappropriate when control, and not full eradication of a disease, is the objective. Since this will almost always be the case, a different strategy will generally be required:

> Control implies sustained high immunization levels in whole populations, which implies in turn unceasing vaccination work in the hamlets and wards where new-born susceptibles accumulate year by year. There can be no decisive victory in a control campaign, and, as a corollary, it makes no sense for vaccinators who need widespread public acceptance and understanding to fall upon the public as upon prey. The public must feel itself a willing subject. (Greenough 1995, p. 643)

And Anne-Emmanuelle Birn reminds us of a doubt expressed by WHO's Director-General at the time smallpox eradication was declared:

> Yet in 1980, WHO's Director-General Halfdan Mahler portended such a less-than-heroic appraisal by declaring: *Important lessons can be learned from smallpox eradication – but the idea that we should single out other diseases for worldwide eradication is not among them. That idea is tempting but illusory.* (Birn 2011)

Mahler's concern, that Birn underwrites in part, was that targeting eradication would divert attention and resources from the structural and economic roots of ill health, and from the commitment to strengthening primary health care that Mahler advocated.

The Expanded Programme of Immunization (1974–)

In May 1974, as the smallpox campaign was entering its final stages, the WHA adopted a Resolution formally establishing an Expanded Programme of Immunization (EPI). Resolution 27.57 recommended Member States to 'develop or maintain immunization and surveillance programmes against some or all of the following diseases: diphtheria, pertussis, tetanus, measles, poliomyelitis, tuberculosis, smallpox and others, where applicable, according to the epidemiological situation in their respective countries'. The Resolution also requested the Director-General (among other things) 'to intensify at all levels of the Organization its activities pertaining to the development of immunization programmes, especially for the developing countries; to assist Member States (i) in developing suitable programmes by providing technical advice on the use of vaccines and (ii) in assuring the availability of good-quality vaccines at reasonable cost; to study the possibilities of providing from international sources and agencies an increased supply of vaccines, equipment and transport and developing local competence to produce vaccines at the national level' (World Health Assembly 1974).

The support of UNICEF was sought, and collaboration formalised at the 1975 meeting of the UNICEF-WHO Joint Committee on Health Policy. The Report of this meeting states that:

> It is of paramount importance that the major effort in the Programme must come from the individual countries concerned. This is for many reasons, one of the most important being that, once established, the national programmes will have to continue into the indefinite future on a regular basis. In the meantime it should be emphasized that the Programme will develop gradually and will expand as more experience in the field is gained and as countries build up their ability to keep a permanent programme going. (UNICEF/WHO 1975)

Initial emphasis was thus going to be on advising and assisting those countries that requested help in developing their immunisation programmes. A series of regional seminars was to be organised at which the necessary steps would be explained to national delegates. The first of these was held in Kumasi, Ghana, in November 1974.

At the 29th WHA, in early 1976, the first year's progress was reviewed. The Director-General's progress report noted that in countries of the African, Latin American, and South-East Asian regions, of the 80 million children born each year only some four million per year were being effectively immunised (World Health Assembly 1976). 'The main objective of this programme is to increase this number as rapidly as possible'. WHO's immediate target was to help countries 'expand the coverage of their immunization programmes. This expansion may be geographical, social, or technical (i.e. in the number of antigens employed)' (World Health Assembly 1976).

The argument was that immunisation had often been neglected because decision-makers in many developing countries were not convinced of its cost-effectiveness. Planning immunisation programmes, it was argued, should start from demographics and disease epidemiology (although in reality epidemiological data were scarce in much of the world), and then move on to assess resources available, forms of organisation, and (socio-cultural) aspects of acceptability. In many countries the view was that, as the smallpox campaign came to an end, financial and human resources invested in it would be transferrable. But at the same time it was also stressed that immunisation should be integrated into basic health services as far as possible.

The significance of this emphasis on integration with primary health care derives from another development taking place at the same time. In 1975 WHO and UNICEF had jointly produced another report entitled 'Alternative Approaches to Meeting Basic Health Care Needs in Developing Countries'. This report, which was profoundly to influence WHO thinking in the following years, was critical of 'vertical' programmes focusing on specific diseases whilst ignoring the 'poverty, squalor and ignorance' that were the real source of ill health in the developing world (Cueto 2004). Drawing on 'Alternative Approaches', Mahler proposed the goal of 'Health for all by the year 2000' at the 1976 WHA. Mahler's thinking helped pave the way for the conference on primary health care that took place in Alma-Ata, Kazakhstan, in September 1978. The Declaration of Alma-Ata, affirmed by the conference, emphasised the importance of health for socioeconomic development and criticised reliance on sophisticated technologies. Primary health care, making use of lay health personnel, encouraging community participation, and integrated with other aspects of development, was to form the cornerstone of public health. The 1979 WHA endorsed the declaration and agreed that primary health care was the key to attaining an acceptable level of health for all.

WHO documents from the early years of EPI continually reaffirm that immunisation should be seen as part of, and not distinct from, primary health care. For example, introducing EPI at a meeting organised by the African region in 1976, the Regional Director for Africa told delegates:

> . . . you must not forget at any time that the programme is above all a national programme integrated into the socioeconomic development of each country. *This activity should be carried out within the national health services structure. The expanded programme on immunization is to be included in the concept of primary health care, basic health measures, and integrated rural development.* (Italics added) (WHO African Region 1976)

It did not take long for dissenting voices to make themselves heard, however. In 1979, Julia Walsh and the Rockefeller Foundation's Kenneth Warren, writing in the *New England Journal of Medicine*, argued that however laudable, the Alma-Ata declaration was unrealistic. The costs of providing clean water, nutritional supplements, and even the most basic primary health care for the world's population could never be met. Walsh and Warren introduced the concept of 'selective primary health care' (Walsh and Warren 1979). Attention and resources should be focused on the most serious diseases, and specifically on those for which simple and effective technologies of prevention or control were available. On this basis they classified diseases into 'high', 'medium', and 'low' priorities. The 'high' category included diarrhoeal diseases, measles, whooping cough, malaria, and neonatal tetanus, the 'medium' category polio, respiratory infections, tuberculosis, and hookworm, whilst in the 'low' category were leprosy, diphtheria, and leishmaniasis. Selective primary health care would then emphasise measles and DPT vaccination, tetanus toxoid for pregnant women, encouragement of long-term breastfeeding, chloroquine for young children in malaria-infested areas, and oral rehydration packets.

Whilst many saw the concept of selective primary health care as a betrayal of the Alma-Ata ideals (Berman 1982; Gish 1982), it corresponded to emphasis within EPI on the use of specific antigens, realistic planning, and quantifiable indicators of progress.

Describing the EPI its Director, RH Henderson, presented it as 'an essential element within WHO's strategy to achieve health for all by the year 2000' (Henderson 1984). Immunisation coverage of children had therefore been included among the indicators that WHO would use to monitor the success of its strategy at the global level. Improvement of national, regional, and global information systems—showing the progress that had been made—was therefore critical. Henderson notes that 'Substantial improvements have occurred between 1978 and 1981 in completing the information available concerning the three principal indices used to monitor progress in the EPI: incidence of the target diseases, immunization coverage, and quality of the vaccines in use.'

Newly available information showed indeed that more and more countries were establishing or extending their immunisation programmes. Giant strides were being taken. For example, Colombia, where in 1975 only 9% of children under 1 year had been immunised with DPT, succeeded in raising coverage to 75% by 1989 (Cueto 2004). This was achieved with active political support and the mobilization of hundreds of teachers, priests, policemen, and Red Cross volunteers. Nevertheless, for critics EPI remained a betrayal of Alma-Ata ideals. For those who held to these ideals, a high level of immunisation coverage was not an appropriate measure of progress in health care. The criteria against which progress had to be judged were the overall adequacy of the healthcare system, popular satisfaction with that system, and community influence over it (Newell 1988). Judged in this way, a successful immunisation programme could even be counterproductive:

> The accounts which are now becoming available from Africa and Asia of the destructive effects at the district and peripheral levels of the health system by processes such as

preferential field allowances to workers participating in vertical EPI programmes are so dramatic that they cannot be ignored. (Newell 1988)

These few critical voices notwithstanding, immunisation programmes have become increasingly central to public health policy over the past 20 years. At the same time vaccination coverage remains the key metric of progress in all official public health fora.

The Child Survival Revolution and Universal Childhood Immunisation (1982–1990)

In 1982, UNICEF's new Executive Director, Harvard-trained lawyer and economist James Grant, announced an initiative called the Child Survival Revolution. Its goal was to promote child health and survival through the use of a few simple and inexpensive medical technologies: growth monitoring, oral rehydration therapy (ORT), breastfeeding, and immunisation (often referred to collectively by the acronym GOBI). A 1984 Conference entitled 'Protecting the World's Children', held at the Rockefeller Foundation's Bellagio Conference Centre, shifted attention specifically to childhood diseases that could be prevented through immunisation. The result was a programme called Universal Childhood Immunization (UCI), and this became the core of the Child Survival Revolution. A clear goal was set: to immunise 80% of the world's children by 1990 (Justice 2000a). With this, UNICEF became a major player in the health field. Not only did some commentators see this as a direct challenge to the role of WHO, but there were clear differences in the preferred strategies of the two organisations. Whilst WHO Director-General (Halfdan Mahler) was deeply committed to the strengthening of primary healthcare services, his UNICEF counterpart, James Grant, emphasised a more 'vertical' attack on vaccine-preventable diseases. Still, there was general agreement that collaboration was essential if the necessary resources and political commitments were to be secured. Judith Justice has explained how the child survival concept was framed with the vagaries of US budgetary politics in mind. 'Gaining active support from U.S. constituents is one way in which child survival was unique, as foreign aid is rarely a priority issue with members of Congress or their constituents. And yet, non-governmental organisations (NGOs) were able to mobilize Americans to use traditional lobbying techniques to succeed in convincing their representatives to support child survival.' (Justice 2000a). It was the grassroots support for Child Survival that led to Congress allocating additional funds to UNICEF and providing funding both for USAID- and US-based NGOs, to be used in support of childhood vaccination.

The institutions and individuals involved with the child survival initiative (which included, in addition to WHO and UNICEF, the Rockefeller Foundation and Robert McNamara, former President of the World Bank) then established a Task Force for Child Survival that would help accelerate immunisation efforts and coordinate support. Established in 1984, the Task Force was located in Atlanta, Georgia, and headed by William Foege, one of the architects of the smallpox eradication campaign.

The Child Survival Revolution culminated in the 1990 World Summit for Children, which was organised by UNICEF and took place in New York in September of that year. Explaining the rationale of the Summit, UNICEF emphasised that it would 'engage the attention and political commitment of leaders, and so give the health and well-being of children a greater priority on political agendas'. By identifying a set of achievable goals, to be achieved by the year 2000, the Summit would keep child survival on the political agenda and would galvanise public support:

> If such goals were few in number, realistic, and addressed to universal concerns, then they could be extremely powerful levers for improving the lives of children over the next ten years. The evidence for this is the highly effective use which has been made of the goal of universal immunization by 1990 (helping to lift immunization coverage from approximately 10% in 1980 to almost 70% by 1989). (UNICEF 1990)

A limited number of goals, widely publicised and acknowledged, agreed to by world leaders, a significant decade and target date: these would be powerful advocacy tools. Of course there were already various sets of goals, but they had for the most part been too detailed and had lacked the power to capture the attention of world leaders. The document goes on to note that:

> Despite the progress made in raising immunization levels from some 10% in 1980 to nearly 70% in 1989, thereby saving the lives of some 6000 children daily, approximately 7000 children still die daily because of vaccine-preventable diseases. The Summit in late September is a compelling impetus for countries with lagging immunization programmes and weak infrastructures to strengthen and accelerate their efforts to achieve Universal Child Immunization by the end of 1990, so that the Head of State/Government will not be in the position of reporting 'failure' when the Summit convenes. (UNICEF 1990)

The health-related goals for the 1990s, set out by UNICEF, included 'Maintenance of a high level of immunisation coverage (at least 85% of children under one year of age) against DPT, BCG, measles, polio and TT', a reduction by 95% in measles deaths and reduction by 90% of measles cases by 1995, compared to pre-immunisation levels, as 'a major step to the global eradication of measles in the longer run', and 'Global eradication of polio by the year 2000' (UNICEF 1990).

UNICEF's Executive Director, James Grant, believed that an event like the Children's Summit would sensitise all heads of state and leaders of governments to the needs of children in their countries (Justice 2000a). Attendance at the Summit seemed to justify his belief. Judith Justice explains that: 'Many national leaders had been personally involved in media campaigns in their countries, appearing on TV and radio, attending immunization sessions and being photographed for posters showing the President or First Lady immunizing children. Thus child immunization was politically attractive at the national level, as well as internationally.' (Justice 2000a).

Whatever its achievements, UNICEF's Child Survival Revolution, and its emphasis on GOBI, provoked alternative interpretations, just as EPI had done. Whatever the value of simple technologies in promoting child health, the way in which the campaign worked in practice undermined local initiatives and competences. Whereas it was perfectly possible for parents to produce oral rehydration mixtures (salt, sugar, water) in their own homes, or to agree among themselves about the importance of breastfeeding, national campaigns did not encourage such initiatives. Rather, media campaigns urged parents to purchase prepackaged rehydration mixtures, and although breastfeeding was encouraged, it was done so (in the words of a contemporary critic):

> . . . with slogans coined outside the affected communities, possibly by the same foreign advertising agencies that had previously sold infant formula and bottle feeding. Immunization, dependent still on a 'cold chain' and considerable logistical preparation, continues to come from 'the top down' but now in massive and possibly unrepeatable campaigns. Little is done to build confidence in people's ability to do positive things about health together, where they live, rather attention is systematically turned toward the 'center' from which wisdom about the breast, magic salts and vaccine issue. (Wisner 1988, p. 964)

Peter Basch drew attention years ago to a disjuncture between international discourse and political opinion at the national level, such that 'some health authorities comment privately that while it is hardly possible to vote openly against such humanitarian resolutions, they and their governments retain a skeptical attitude' (Basch 1994, pp. 45–6). He also felt that willingness to speak out was growing. Thus:

> The Minister of Health of a large African country, speaking at a conference on international health in 1989, criticized GOBI . . . as an unwelcome diversion from the thrust of national health care policies. A senior educator from a large South Asian nation characterized Child Survival and GOBI as poorly conceived mass campaigns and simplistic approaches to complex problems. He claimed that poor people were 'the target of magic bullets fired by foreign bureaucrats who have missed the target'. (Basch 1994, pp. 45–6)

Polio eradication (1988–)

Despite outgoing Director-General Mahler's earlier warning, the 1988 WHA endorsed the UNICEF goal of 'Eradication of Polio by the year 2000'. Historian William Muraskin has provided an invaluable account of the events leading up to this new emphasis in immunisation policy (Muraskin 2012).

In 1980 a meeting took place at the National Institutes of Health in Bethesda, Maryland. Drawing its inspiration from the smallpox eradication campaign, the meeting was intended to identify future eradication targets. Two of the principal architects of smallpox eradication, Frank Fenner and DA Henderson, argued that there simply were no feasible eradication targets. The organisers of the meeting were undeterred. It was a matter of ideology, of faith, rooted in opposition to post-Alma-Ata emphasis on strengthening primary health and belief in eradication. It was this small group of influential American public health experts, committed to eradication, who drove things along. It was essential that the smallpox campaign be followed up: it mattered less which disease was targeted. Measles and polio were identified as the most promising candidates, and in 1983 a symposium on polio control took place at Pan American Health Organization (PAHO) Headquarters in Washington DC. Virtually no speakers at the meeting argued in favour of eradication. Polio was not a major public health concern in the developing world, and 'control' was a more appropriate goal. Nevertheless, thanks to the efforts of a small group of men, a mere 5 years later the WHA was to endorse polio eradication. In 1985 Ciro de Quadros secured the commitment of the PAHO Council to eradication of polio in the Americas by 1990. His objective, according to Muraskin, was to use polio eradication as a means of strengthening health systems, and specifically EPI programmes, in Latin American countries. (This was despite the fact that the head of EPI at WHO Headquarters, Ralph Henderson, was not supportive of a polio eradication campaign (Muraskin 2012, p. 37).) DA Henderson agreed to act as technical advisor to the PAHO programme, believing that although global eradication was not feasible, eradication in the Americas was. Moreover, such a goal, he believed, would attract political support for improved disease surveillance systems. Just 2 years later, and long before eradication had been achieved in the Americas, De Quadros and a group of CDC colleagues published an article arguing for global eradication (Hinman et al. 1987). A year later, Foege's Task Force for Child Survival organised a high-level meeting in Talloires (France) to establish global health priorities for the 1990s. Foege and UNICEF Executive Director James Grant made clear their support for global polio eradication. Even outgoing Director-General Halfdan Mahler seems to have been convinced by experience in the Americas, despite continuing resistance from the head of EPI (Muraskin 2012, pp. 54–6). In the 'Declaration of Talloires', resulting from the meeting, polio eradication headed the list of global health goals for the 1990s. The WHA Resolution followed just 2 months later.

The global polio eradication campaign adopted a four-pronged strategy. It was to consist of achieving and maintaining high coverage with at least three doses of oral polio vaccine (OPV), providing supplementary doses of OPV to all children aged less than 5 years during national immunisation days (NIDs), surveillance for all cases of acute flaccid paralysis (AFP) in children aged less than 15 years and virological examination of stool specimens from each case, and house-to-house OPV 'mop-up' campaigns, targeting areas in which transmission of wild poliovirus persisted. It became apparent that NIDs and the 'mop-up' activities would demand a vast investment of labour.

> In many countries NIDs have been the largest public health activity ever conducted. Based on the number of people needed to operate a polio immunization post during a NID, and the average number of children immunized per day at such a post, it is estimated that at least 10 million people have participated in polio NIDs at some point in the eradication initiative. (Aylward and Linkins 2005)

Vaccinators' tasks were relatively simple. They would have to select and arrange a local immunisation site, organise the children for immunisation, give each child two drops of the OPV, record the number of children immunised, and submit this information together with unused vaccine to a supervisor. It was believed that with half a day of training and continuous supervision these tasks could be carried out by assistants without any formal education.

In 1994 the Americas were declared polio-free. Whilst PAHO experience had been used to show what could be achieved in the rest of the world, some of those involved felt that the commitment of national governments in that region was not paralleled in other WHO regions. It therefore provided an inappropriate model of what might happen elsewhere (Muraskin 2012, p. 73). Even within the Americas the programme had consequences that differed widely from country to country. This was the conclusion drawn by three eminent public health specialists on the basis of a 1995 study of the impact of polio eradication (and EPI) in six countries in the Americas:

> The overall conclusion was that polio eradication contributed positively to health systems and helped generate a 'culture of prevention' in these middle-income countries with well-established health infrastructures. Most positive was the promotion of social mobilization and intersectoral cooperation, two of the Alma-Ata primary health care goals that have been the most difficult to implement. The Expanded Programme on Immunization strengthened managerial, epidemiological, and laboratory capacity and was an important catalyst for donor coordination. The management, laboratory, and surveillance systems helped in measles elimination activities. (Taylor et al. 1997)

However, Taylor et al. also pointed to a risk that targeted vertical immunisation programmes could drain resources from other, routine, health services. A detailed study of the origins, evolution, and impact of vertically organised immunisation programmes in Ecuador and El Salvador goes further. It questions not only the impact of the NIDs, so praised by WHO officials, on routine services, but on longer-term rates of coverage (Gloyd et al. 2003). Ecuador, in 1977, had been one of the first countries in Latin America to introduce EPI. A conservative president, elected in 1984, was committed to implementing World Bank structural adjustment policies. Having devoted little attention to social programmes, President Febres Cordero was receptive to a suggestion from the executive director of UNICEF that he introduce a mass immunisation effort. Funded by a US$4 million grant from USAID, this Program for Reducing Maternal and Infant Mortality had increasing polio and DPT immunisation and increasing ORT usage among its specific objectives. A parallel administrative structure was established to run the programme, staffed by international experts and senior Ministry of Health (MoH) staff seconded at much higher than normal salaries. 'This new unit affected the structure and organization of the MoH, and it marked the beginning of a downtrend in the ministry's political importance, resources, and ability to provide services' (Gloyd et al. 2003, p. 117). Seven NID campaigns took place in Ecuador, supported by massive media promotion, before USAID support ended, in 1989. Reviewing coverage data for DPT3 and measles immunisation, as well as reported measles incidence from 1979 to 1993, this study concludes that the vast investment in NIDs had had little long-term effect. When support from USAID ended, both administrative organisation and routine programmes had difficulty in filling the gap created. Immediately after the intensive immunisation programmes ended numbers of measles cases rose to higher levels than they had been before the programmes started. Moreover the cost per vaccination dose in the Ecuador campaigns was nearly three times higher than for vaccinations provided through routine services (Gloyd et al. 2003, p. 125).

Despite enormous progress, and a drastic reduction in cases of polio reported, the initial objective—eradication by the year 2000—proved unattainable. In 2007, after the expenditure of US$4.5 billion (double the amount initially estimated), it was noted that the number of cases reported globally in 2006 was higher than in any of the previous 6 years. In Afghanistan, India, Nigeria, and Pakistan, polio remained endemic, and travellers were soon found to have exported it to other countries (Lahariya 2007). A funding deficit was reported: the resources available were not going to be adequate. Lahariya notes that in the areas in which polio still occurs 'the hurdles to be faced are all different, and eradication may not be achieved by the same strategies'. Many critics go further than this, arguing that the global polio eradication campaign was a mistake from the start. In their view eradication enthusiasts had thought too little about possible impact on routine immunisation services or the demands polio eradication would place on understaffed health services. Critique appears to be most scathing in India, and Muraskin devotes a whole chapter of his book to the arguments of the 'Indian dissenters'. For one thing, the country has other health priorities. For another, Indian critics resent the oft-stated view that the country's failure to eliminate polio is due to a lack of 'political will' when, in their view, India has conscientiously followed WHO advice (Sathyamala et al. 2005).

Developing and introducing new vaccines (1990–)

The growing influence of neoliberal thinking from the early 1980s onwards had major consequences for international health policy generally and for vaccination specifically. The view that the private sector had to be more explicitly involved in international health policy formulation was becoming increasingly influential. This was partly for ideological reasons and partly in acknowledgement of the UN system's lack of resources and what some governments perceived as its lack of effectiveness (Buse and Walt 2000). If the world's health problems were adequately to be addressed in the era of globalisation, then it would be essential to involve a greater variety of stakeholders, industry in particular. Partnerships involving international agencies, donors, and industry would not only introduce additional resources, they could also provide a means of bringing the skills and expertise available in industry more effectively to bear on the health problems of the developing world. A wide variety of global public–private partnerships (GPPPs) emerged, many of them aimed at development and production of drugs and vaccines needed in the developing world.

At the 1985 Conference of the Task Force of Child Survival Foege cited findings of an inquiry among EPI programme managers on what they would want if they had the power to design an ideal vaccine:

> (T)hey would develop a multi-antigen vaccine (that is containing all antigens in a single injection), that would: (1) provide life-long immunity with a single dose (2) have no short-term or long-term adverse reactions; (3) be inexpensive; (4) be easily administered without costly equipment or techniques by relatively untrained workers; (5) be stable at tropical temperatures for months, or even years; (6) be efficacious at any time after birth. (Foege 1985, cited in Muraskin 1998)

Co-sponsored by the UNDP, WHO, the World Bank, the Rockefeller Foundation, and UNICEF (the same actors who had been involved in UCI), the Children's Vaccine Initiative (CVI) was established in 1990. Working together with private industry, in a way that WHO was prohibited by its charter from doing, the CVI would, as a major objective, stimulate development of new and better vaccines (Muraskin 1998). For this cooperation with the pharmaceutical industry was essential. Through the 1990s a variety of tensions emerged, however. One of the CVI's early goals was facilitating development of a more heat-stable polio vaccine. The sensitivity to heat of the OPV meant that its transport necessitated establishment of long and complex 'cold chains', the maintenance of which caused endless problems. Industry was persuaded to cooperate in developing a more heat-resistant vaccine. It invested resources on the assumption that, when available, the new polio vaccine would be adopted on a large scale. But when, later, leaders of EPI and the polio eradication initiative decided that such a vaccine was not needed, and would not be used, industry was, unsurprisingly, frustrated. The public sector was coming to seem an untrustworthy partner. Tensions also emerged between European and American donors to WHO and UNICEF. Some Europeans donors, especially the Dutch and Nordic countries, felt that CVI was too American a project: too focused on finding technological solutions for health problems in developing countries. There were fears that commercial interests would dominate CVI (Muraskin 1998, pp. 152–3). In the event the CVI failed in its attempts to generate harmonious relationships between stakeholders, failed to establish an agreed and visible role for itself, and failed in its attempts to stimulate new vaccine development. It gradually shifted its attention to new vaccine introduction: a topic of great interest to industry, and one neglected by an EPI leadership that had little enthusiasm for adding to the costs and difficulties of the programme (Muraskin 1998). Disagreements between the CVI's principal sponsors proved unbridgeable and led to its closure in 1999. However, for organisations looking to create a global alliance in its place, in which industry had to be a participant, stimulating new vaccine introduction became an ever more central objective.

At the end of the new millennium, CVI was overtaken by the Global Alliance for Vaccines and Immunisation (GAVI) and the accompanying multimillion dollar Global Fund for Children's Vaccines.

The public–private venture known as GAVI was announced to the public at the 2000 World Economic Forum held in Davos. GAVI's strategy, inspired by CVI, involved improving access to sustainable immunisation services, expanding the use of all cost-effective vaccines, accelerating the introduction of new vaccines, speeding up efforts to create new vaccines, and making immunisation a central part of assessing international development efforts. Its founding partners included WHO, UNICEF, the World Bank, the Bill and Melinda Gates Children's Vaccine Program, the Rockefeller Foundation, the International Federation of Pharmaceutical Manufacturers' Associations (IFPMA), and some national governments. GAVI, now known as the GAVI Alliance, is discussed in more detail in Chapter 3. Although the most important public–private partnership in the area of vaccination, it is far from being the only one. Others established at roughly the same time include the Hookworm Vaccine Initiative, the International AIDS Vaccine Initiative (IAVI), the Leishmania Vaccine Initiative, and the Malaria Vaccine Initiative (MVI).

Writing in 2000, Buse and Walt saw these partnerships as potentially benefitting all stakeholders: industry, for example, would gain greater access to global health governance, whilst the UN system would gain much-needed resources. On the other hand, they also foresaw potential pitfalls, including declining influence of developing country governments (with less of a voice in the management of GPPPs than in UN organisations) and lack of transparency and accountability (Buse and Walt 2000). Wheeler and Berkeley, themselves at the time associated with two of these initiatives, explained that they functioned as 'social venture capitalists', identifying and supporting promising projects, and looking to stimulate their production and distribution at affordable prices (Wheeler and Berkley 2001). 'Typically,' they write, 'the partnerships expect that collaborating companies will ultimately manufacture and distribute the final product, providing advantaged access to the developing world through lower pricing and other means' (Wheeler and Berkley 2001, p. 731). To this end, and to enable the companies to make a profit, control over intellectual property rights and appropriate licensing agreements become crucial. So too do good working relationships with established international organisations: IAVI, for example, rapidly established good links with UNAIDS and the World Bank. Joanna Chataway and her colleagues have been studying two of these initiatives, IAVI and the MVI, over a number of years. They show how the two organisations have evolved rather differently (Chataway et al. 2010). IAVI has tended to see itself as a 'virtual pharmaceutical company', and now has its own laboratories in New York. However, from its origins in 1996 it has always devoted attention also to outreach work: to working closely with national governments and community organisations in developing countries themselves. The MVI, which was established in 1999 with funding from the BMGF, has tended to focus more exclusively on vaccine development. It has also worked very closely with the pharmaceutical industry, especially GlaxoSmithKline (GSK). As a GSK malaria vaccine works its way through clinical trials, with success, the role of the MVI may be changing.

All these organisations are committed principally to the development and introduction of new vaccines, deploying a range of policy mechanisms to that end. That and how they do so will become clearer from subsequent chapters of this book.

Perhaps unsurprisingly, GAVI strategy and priorities are also subject to considerable criticism. Critics are concerned by the organisation's emphasis on the introduction of expensive new vaccines in countries which lack the resources to continue vaccination once GAVI funding ends. Organisations like Oxfam and Médecins Sans Frontières (Doctors without Borders; MSF) are critical of pharmaceutical company influence on GAVI decision-making (Boseley 2011).

International health in the 20th century: lessons from history

We have charted the history of 20th century public health, and of immunisation as one of its most vital tools, in terms of a series of initiatives that have built one on the other. Each of them has been contested, with conflicting perspectives on one or the other themselves reflecting the ideological conflicts and struggles for influence (and for independence) that marked the century's political history. Thus Peruvian historian of public health Marcos Cueto sees 20th century international health in terms of two distinctive configurations of assumptions, built either around a sense of disease as a consequence of social and economic underdevelopment and inequality or around a sense of disease as a natural phenomenon in need of technological solutions.

Cueto's two paths equate, in effect, with (comprehensive) primary health care and selective primary health care, respectively. In the case of the first:

> The combination can be summarized as the crisis of the Cold War, the prominence of Mahler at the WHO, the utopian goal of 'Health for All', and an unspecific methodology. The combination in the case of selective primary health care was neo-liberalism, the leadership of Grant as head of UNICEF, the more modest goal of a 'children's revolution', and GOBI interventions. (Cueto 2004)

Immunisation programmes do not correspond in any essential way to one or other of these approaches. For one thing, the rhetoric with which they have been explained and justified, and with which resources have been mobilized, has drawn on one or the other, depending on circumstances. For some, on some occasions, immunisation programmes were to be an essential element in the strengthening of basic healthcare provision, whilst for others, or on other occasions, they would only divert attention from the structural causes of ill health and health inequality. For another thing, and more importantly, the consequences of globally orchestrated immunisation programmes are not the same everywhere. As some public health researchers warned in the 1990s, the positive effects of the polio eradication campaign for health services in the Americas was unlikely to be replicated in Africa. And even within the Americas, as Taylor et al. discovered, there were significant differences in the effects of the campaign, and EPI, on middle-income countries with well-organised health systems on the one hand, and poor countries with weakly organised health systems on the other.

The logic underlying the succession of global immunisation programmes discussed here is essentially the logic of international politics. Each was crafted in the light of the balance of political interests of its time, shaped in order to mobilise support from a variety of sources, and to sustain the commitment of a range of public and private donors.

> They help mobilise collective energies behind collective goals, and they help sustain the hope that the aims can be achieved. They project an image of possible and intrinsically beneficial public health programmes. The initiatives were formulated at different times in response to somewhat different ideologies and configurations of power. (Hardon and Blume 2005, p. 353)

Mobilising the resources required and securing the commitment of major stakeholders have made sensitivity to dominant ideologies and configurations of power essential. Since these have changed dramatically since the 1970s, the assumptions underlying international health policy today are not the same as those of 30 or 40 years ago. As later chapters will show, major stakeholders have become both more numerous and more heterogeneous. They now include not only national governments (both as consumers of vaccines and in some cases as donors), but also suppliers of vaccines (principally, although not exclusively, the multinational pharmaceutical industry), NGOs, and major philanthropic organisations such as the BMGF. The changing political, social, and economic context of international health policy has also led to changes in the way in which the success of programmes is understood (Birn 2009). Despite critique addressed to each of the initiatives discussed here, immunisation programmes have become increasingly central to international public health. Three sets of assumptions seem to underpin current investment in children's health today. In the course of three or four decades these assumptions have become so taken-for-granted that they are rarely, if ever, held up for debate.

Increasing reliance on technology

Introducing their concept of 'selective primary health care' in 1979, Walsh and Warren presented what had been agreed at Alma-Ata as an unrealistic ideal: 'The goal set at Alma-Ata is above reproach, yet its large and laudable scope makes it unattainable. . . . ' (Walsh and Warren 1979, p. 145). Selective primary health care was presented as an 'interim' strategy, designed to secure the greatest value for money, in terms of children's lives saved. The focus was to be on specific diseases that caused high mortality and morbidity, and for which inexpensive technologies of control were available. The simple technologies they listed (including measles and DPT immunisation, breastfeeding and ORT) were not very different from those subsequently promoted by UNICEF's Child Survival Revolution and known by the acronym GOBI. Walsh and Warren did not address the question of where these simple technologies were to come from. Within a handful of years, critics of the Child Survival Revolution could focus precisely on this. Parents might have been taught how to prepare oral rehydration solutions in their own homes, whereas in practice they were being advised to purchase prepackaged mixtures (Wisner 1988). To be sure, educating parents, persuading people to change their behaviour, takes time and effort. The benefits of health education campaigns take time to realise and are not always easy to measure. The costs are soon apparent whilst the gains, if translated into money terms, are not. Moreover, no-one stands to make a direct profit from teaching parents how to mix salt, sugar, and water for treating diarrhoea. Commercial ORT packages, however, are a different matter. Vaccines too are of course commercial commodities, and by the 1980s the bulk of them were supplied by profit-making corporations. Technological approaches to controlling disease have the advantage of promising a clear and measurable solution to a complex problem. They are also potentially profitable.

In the 1980s a number of fundamental changes occurred in the conceptual underpinnings of international health policy. These changes have their roots in the rise of neoliberal thinking, involving privatisation and free reign to market forces, that the World Bank made a condition of its loans (which were becoming increasingly important in the health sector). In this new international regime countries were obliged to dismantle protectionist barriers to the free flow of capital and goods. In the early years of EPI, support for local vaccine production and for the establishment of local and regional markets was stressed as a policy objective. Gradually reference to this goal faded. The pharmaceutical industry was coming to be seen as a vital partner in developing international immunisation policy, and this industry was increasingly dominated by a small number of large firms seeking global markets. It was becoming expedient, if not essential, to acknowledge their interests in extending their markets and recouping investments in developing new vaccines. The public–private partnerships that were established from the 1990s onwards, the new policy instruments (including the Advance Market Commitment and the International Finance Facility for Immunisation) that were designed, were intended to bring industrial resources and expertise to bear on the objectives of public health. They also gave industry growing influence on the formulation of those objectives.

The multinational vaccine industry is now an influential participant in global decision-making (although its structure is changing as developing country manufacturers extend their market shares). A consequence is that the rapid introduction of new vaccines has become a priority alongside control of diseases of acknowledged public health importance. As discussed in more detail in Chapter 4, delays in the introduction of new vaccines then come to be seen as problematic. Thus the 2005 WHO/UNICEF strategy document quoted earlier refers to the slow introduction of hepatitis B vaccine, which had been recommended for routine use in 1992. It goes on to note that 'A similar time lag is unfortunately now being experienced with Haemophilus influenzae type b vaccine, for which global coverage remains low at 22%' (WHO/UNICEF 2005). Something needed to be done.

The growing self-evidence of a global perspective

Technological approaches to complex health problems appeal to policy-makers: perhaps above all to those at the global level, furthest removed from cultural and social specificities. Reviewing the history of public health in colonial and post-colonial India, for example, Amrith explains that 'The very attraction of a techno-centric approach to public health was that it appeared to detach WHO from the need to intervene deeply, in matters of "culture" or social transformation' (Amrith 2006, p. 17). Amrith's study deals with the period up to 1965. Since that time technological possibilities have multiplied and WHO now shares responsibility for international health with a variety of other organisations. Yet his conclusion has lost little of its force in today's globalising era. The consequences of globalisation for immunisation are not wholly captured by reference to the changing structure of the vaccine market or the growing influence of multinational manufacturers. No less significant is a decline in the authority of nation states and their governments. We see it in areas such as the Caucasus, where the status of regions such as Abkhazia and South Ossetia is internationally disputed, or in the Middle East. But questions about sovereignty go beyond controversy regarding national boundaries or statehood. The wrangling in many European countries regarding the extent to which they should or are willing to transfer powers to European institutions offers a different kind of example. The implications of these debates about national sovereignty, and about the balance of responsibilities between national governments and international organisations, differ from one area of policy to another. Acknowledgement that the growing scale of international mobility has rendered national boundaries increasingly permeable to all kinds of pathogens has given a legitimacy to global governance in the public health field that is not paralleled in, for example, educational policy or taxation.

The International Health Regulations provide a good illustration of what we mean. From the mid-19th century onwards, states subscribed to international agreements intended to protect their borders against the introduction of infectious pathogens via trade and migration. Although these International Health Regulations (IHRs) have regularly been amended, their core is an obligation on governments to inform WHO about outbreaks of infectious disease of likely international significance. Until recently these requirements related only to specific named diseases (so that after eradication smallpox was removed from the list). By the 1990s the existing IHRs were coming to seem inadequate, partly due to the emergence of new infectious diseases and partly due to the failure of many governments to comply with the regulations (Fidler and Gostin 2006). Work on a new radically revised set of regulations began, hastened by the outbreak of severe acute respiratory syndrome (SARS) in 2003. The revised IHRs, adopted by the WHA in 2005, are intended to facilitate a public health response to the international spread of disease in ways compatible with state sovereignty and human rights, and which minimise disruptions of international trade. The obligation on governments to notify WHO of events that may lead to a public health emergency of international importance remains. But a number of important modifications were introduced. One was that the restriction to named diseases was removed. The 2005 Regulations refer to an 'illness or medical condition, irrespective of origin or source, that presents or could present significant harm to humans' (World Health Organization 2008a). A second was an extension in the surveillance that governments were required to carry out. Previously, surveillance had only been required at points of entry and exit (harbours, airports, and so on). The new Regulations require surveillance of national territories as a whole—although without addressing the question of how these surveillance capacities are to be established in poor countries (Calain 2006a,b). The third major change is that WHO is now allowed to make use not only of notifications provided by governments, but of any other source of information (mass media, the internet, information provided by NGOs) it regards as relevant. WHO must then only seek 'verification' from the government concerned. In this way the likelihood that a government may fail to comply because of fears that trade or tourism will be affected is bypassed. 'In short,' conclude Fidler and Gostin, 'the information and verification provisions privilege global health governance over state sovereignty' (Fidler and Gostin 2006, p. 90). Some commentators, reflecting on successes in tackling emerging pandemic diseases such as SARS, thus argue that *only* through centrally (i.e. globally) planned and managed initiatives, the subordination of national responsibilities and jurisdictions to a global authority (in which the private sector is also represented) can the spread of infectious diseases effectively be combated (Fidler 2004). It is in line with this perspective that WHO and UNICEF propose the 'global strategy' discussed earlier in this chapter.

The growing importance of targets

Targets have played a crucial role in relation to each of the initiatives discussed here. They have ranged from the very general, like 'Health for all by the year 2000', to the very specific, such as UNICEF's goals for the 1990s (including, for example, 'a reduction by 95% in measles deaths and reduction by 90% of measles cases by 1995, compared to pre-immunization levels') (World Health Organization 2008b). As UNICEF pointed out in explaining the need for its 1990 Summit, a small number of realistic goals could be 'powerful advocacy tools throughout the decade' (World Health Organization 2008b).

Targets have become important for essentially political reasons. This holds true at all levels, from that of global organisations to that of the community health centre (Das et al. 2000). Participants at all levels experience the need to show that progress is being made. At the global level, targets have become essential to resource mobilization and to maintaining the commitment of the world's political leaders. They also provide an end point against which progress can be demonstrated, provided appropriate data are collected regularly. Surveillance data, demonstrating progress (or in the case of epidemics, failure), are essential in convincing donors that whilst their money has been well spent there remains a significant distance still to be travelled if targets are to be met. Today, the goals that dominate international debate are the so-called Millennium Development Goals (MDGs). Adopted by all 193 UN Member States in September 2000, the eight MDGs originated from the UN's Millennium Declaration. The Declaration asserts that every individual has the right to dignity, freedom, equality, and a basic standard of living that includes freedom from hunger and violence, and encourages tolerance and solidarity. Of the eight MDGs, three (numbers 4, 5, and 6) address health issues specifically. Thus goal 4 is 'Reduce by two-thirds, between 1990 and 2015, the under-five mortality rate', whilst 5 relates to maternal health and 6 to slowing and then stopping the spread of HIV/AIDS, malaria, and tuberculosis (UN 2010).

Their origins (and the question of 'Why these and not others?') have been fascinatingly described by one of their architects (Vandemoortele 2011). Vandemoortele explains how a group of experts from different UN organisations and the Organisation for Economic Co-operation and Development (OECD) set about extracting a set of targets from the UN's Millennium Declaration. Limits were set. Only targets with 'agreed indicators and with robust data' were to be included. For this reason things like 'the quality of education, the affordability of water, good governance and human rights' were not included, and nor were possible health indicators relating to chronic illness or mental health. Whilst this work was being done in 2000, 1990 was chosen as the baseline year.

This was partly because 'most global targets contained in the Millennium Declaration had their origin in the 1990s at the various world summits and international conferences,' and these had used 1990 as their baseline. It was also because attaining goals such as a two-thirds reduction in infant mortality, or a three-quarters reduction in maternal mortality, within a mere 15 years seemed hopelessly unrealistic. The original intention, Vandemoortele explains, was not that each individual country meet all the targets. Nor were they intended to guide the detailed work of policy-makers or practitioners in the field. They were to play a role in a much more general political and media discourse. 'The primary purpose of the MDGs was precisely to make the dominant narrative a bit more sophisticated by focusing on equitable and sustainable well-being, beyond the narrow domain of economic growth' (Vandemoortele 2011, p. 8). Vandemoortele ends his article with an angry assault on how the MDGs have been 'distorted', i.e. turned into a set of technical prescriptions, whilst what their achievement requires is societal change necessarily driven by local politics and local actors.

In the sense their architects intended the MDG agenda will fail because of the extent to which 'the pattern of progress has been inequitable in the majority of countries'. Indeed empirical research had shown that progress toward the child mortality goal not uncommonly conceals growing mortality differences between rich and poor (Moser et al. 2005).

> Behind each preventable child death, behind each malnourished child, behind each maternal death . . . lies a story of high inequality and deep-seated discrimination. In other words, poverty will be eradicated not by more aid or more growth but by greater equality. (Vandemoortele 2011, p. 18)

However, as Walsh and Warren's influential reformulation of the Alma-Ata goals in terms of an 'interim strategy' of 'selective primary health care' had shown 30 years previously, donor agencies are reluctant to address inequalities within countries. Targets chosen had to reflect the interests, and the preferred strategies, of powerful stakeholders. In WHO and UNICEF's Global Immunisation Vision and Strategy document, with which we opened this chapter, immunisation is presented as a vital tool in achieving the MDGs. This document outlines the assumptions, the vision, and the strategies on which immunisation programmes now rest.

The achievements of immunisation programmes are demonstrated by reference to global increases in coverage (e.g. 'In 2006, global routine coverage with measles vaccine reached 80% for the first time, increasing from 72% in 2000'), reductions in mortality (e.g. 'Between 2000 and 2006, global mortality due to measles was reduced by 68% from an estimated 757 000 deaths in 2000 to

242 000 in 2006'), and aggregate numbers of lives saved (e.g. 'These public health accomplishments helped to prevent nearly 9.2 million measles deaths between 2000 and 2006') (World Health Organization 2008b). The distance still to be travelled (leaving aside the fact that some countries still lack even basic registration of births and deaths), as affirmed at the 61st WHA, which took place in 2008, was to be understood in terms of the numbers of children who were unvaccinated or only partially vaccinated, the large variations in coverage among regions and countries, and the delays with which new vaccines are introduced in much of the world.

In 2008, on the 30th anniversary of the Alma-Ata declaration, Halfdan Mahler (who had retired as WHO Director-General in 1988) addressed the 61st WHA (Mahler 2008). He reminded delegates that primary health care had meant essential health care, based on accepted methods and technology, and made universally accessible at a cost that communities and countries can afford, and in a 'spirit of self-reliance and self-determination' (Mahler 2008). Going on to quote from the Declaration of Alma-Ata, Mahler explained that primary health care includes health education, promotion of proper nutrition, sanitation and an adequate supply of safe water, maternal and child health care, including family planning, immunisation against the major infectious diseases, prevention and control of locally endemic diseases, and provision of essential drugs. Many of these objectives do not sound very different from the health-related MDGs (to which UN Member States recommitted themselves in September 2010). However, the similarity of the goals is deceptive and does not imply any similarity in the actions taken in pursuit of them. Shaped by the very different political configurations of the 21st century, the uses to which they are being put are likely to be very different indeed.

The perspective and structure of the book

Immunologically speaking, the vaccines now in widespread use are very effective. Children who have been fully vaccinated against a disease are unlikely to contract it. But immunology is not the whole story. The contribution that vaccines make to the health of the world's children in practice depends on much more than their effect on the individual recipient's immune system. For one thing, it depends on children's access to immunisation programmes. And this, in turn, depends on how the programmes are organised, on commitment to making them work, from the political level to the level of the village health worker. It depends on a reliable supply of vaccines and on the trust of the community. The current reality is that vaccine coverage is highly unequal, with major variations both between countries and within some individual countries.

This is clearly undesirable, however inadequate a measure of children's welfare vaccine coverage may be. Current strategy involves efforts to extend coverage to children (for example in remote regions or from underprivileged population groups) who have previously not been reached. This is clearly to be welcomed, although it is equally clearly not enough. Our purpose in writing this book is not to assess the extent of progress being made, whether towards the MDGs or any other indicator of progress. What we try to do here is to hold up for examination the assumptions on which immunisation programmes today rest and explore their implications in practice. As this chapter has shown, each step in the evolution of global immunisation policy, from the commitment to smallpox eradication onwards, has attracted criticism. Critique has often been based on a priori approval or disapproval: of 'vertical' approaches to public health, or the effects of the polio eradication campaign, or current emphasis on new vaccine introduction. Yet, as some of the studies quoted in this chapter have shown, the effects of a global programme can differ considerably from one country to another depending, for example, on the organisation and robustness of a health system, or popular trust in it. Our argument will be much in the spirit of Banerjee and Duflo's call to ground the fight against poverty in the knowledge of local people rather than in all-encompassing ideologies (Banerjee and Duflo 2011). Vaccines are powerful tools that will best serve children's health if they are used in ways that respect and gently shift (rather than overwhelm) political and social realities, and local knowledge and concerns.

In Chapter 2 we discuss our perspective in more detail. We suggest that immunisation-in-practice can be conceptualised in terms of a chain, linking the global level, through the national and local levels, to the individual parent whose child is to be immunised. The necessities of immunisation flow along this chain: resources such as money and vaccines, knowledge and expertise, authority and norms, plans, reports, and numbers. Resources, combined with moral zeal, drive the process, but the flows can also be challenged and resisted. Drawing on anthropological discussions, we discuss what happens at the interfaces between these levels. Chapter 3 looks at the changing structure of the global level, analysing how relevant global institutions interact with each other in formulating goals, setting targets, providing resources, and requiring proofs of performance. The different actors draw on distinctive and potentially competing sources of authority. On some occasions the different global actors coordinate and cooperate, on others they conflict and compete. Since the mid-1990s the GAVI has brought an increasing degree of unity, coordination, and coherence to the global level, with as a consequence a growing influence over national policy-making. Chapter 4 poses the question: 'How do global health bodies influence national immunisation policies, and how (conversely) do national policies influence global goals, procedures, and resources?' There is no single answer to either of these questions. Differences in size and wealth, health system dependence on (or independence of) donor resources, political differences in interactions between health and foreign policy, the presence (or not) of a domestic vaccine industry: all play a role. Focusing particularly on the intro-duction of new vaccines, the chapter explores the range of interactions between the global and national levels. In Chapter 5 we focus on national policy-making and the organisation of immunisation programmes. Despite the standardising influence of global policies and objectives, health systems and their governance differ considerably between countries and, in some cases, between regions of the same country. So, as a consequence, do the ways in which immunisation programmers are organised, staffed, funded, and supplied with the resources they need. How, for example, is immunisation integrated with other health and welfare services focused on children, and what difference does their integration or non-integration make in practice? Whilst immunisation is generally organ-ised as a routine practice, on occasion public health systems are confronted by a crisis. How do they cope, and what lasting effects do crisis measures have? Chapter 6 deals with local immunisation practices. Whether understood in terms of improvements in child health or in terms of coverage, the success of an immunisation programme depends ultimately on what happens where health workers, representing the national health system, meet mothers and their chil-dren. Drawing principally on ethnographic studies carried out in two regions of India and in Malawi, in this chapter we focus on activities taking place at the community level, especially during national vaccination days. The chapter examines critically how local health workers in different settings manoeuvre between, or try to reconcile, the often conflicting demands of being responsible for ensuring that targets are met on the one hand, whilst developing a relation-ship of trust with the community on the other.

In the final chapter we discuss the overall argument of the book and its impli-cations. The structure of the book reflects the structure of global health and immunisation policies, in terms of downward flows of resources, plans, and expertise. The targets set globally, the mechanisms prescribed, and the resources provided are informed by a logic that is increasingly shaped by strategic considerations and interests. Actors at lower levels in the system are expected to meet targets, use resources efficiently, and report on their actions. The pressures and the incentives generated throughout the system, reflecting this normative structure of action, encourage reports of success. By contrast, qualitative and quantitative information on failure to meet targets, vaccine-attributable adverse events, failures in the vaccine supply system such as theft or wastage, the difficulties faced by local health workers, and loss of trust tends to be suppressed. It is this suppressed knowledge of local realities that forms the focus of the chapter's concluding section. Looking upwards rather than downwards, would immunisation programmes, and hence global child health, differ were local knowledge and realities permitted to inform national and international policy?

Chapter 2

Concepts and approaches

Stuart Blume, Sidsel Roalkvam,
and Desmond McNeill

Introduction: thinking about globalisation

In Chapter 1 we suggested that new immunisation initiatives build on each
other over time according to a distinctive logic. A key element of that logic is
the growth in authority and influence of a global perspective on public health
generally and on immunisation specifically. This reflects both the rise in
resources available to and through international agencies such as the GAVI
Alliance, and the way in which public health has come to be seen as 'global
health' (Brown et al. 2004). The various initiatives discussed in Chapter 1 also
have a crucial feature in common. All are concerned with effectively delivering
vaccines to children worldwide. Modern vaccines are sophisticated products
based on years of research and development. Before large-scale trials designed
to establish their protective efficacy can begin, they have to be exhaustively
tested in laboratory animals and in small-scale pilot studies. The costs of getting a new vaccine out into the health system these days are estimated at
around US$500–1000 million. Small wonder that today most new vaccines are
developed by a very few giant pharmaceutical companies competing in a global market. It was not always so. Many of the public health laboratories established a century ago had the task of supplying vaccines for national
immunisation programmes. In a few countries of the global North (notably
the Netherlands and the Scandinavian countries) and in many of the global
South this was still the case until quite recently. When the first polio and measles vaccines were being developed, in the 1950s and 1960s, virus strains and
production processes were not protected by patents, and it was not too difficult
for national laboratories to set about developing and producing them (Blume
2005). Like the immunisation programmes discussed in Chapter 1, changes in
the organisation of vaccine development and production over the past few
decades are a consequence of globalisation. If we want to understand how,
today, these sophisticated materials reach the bodies of children in far-flung

villages, we need to do so in the context of today's global world. In order to understand the significance of this context, some concepts from anthropology will be helpful.

Many people think of globalisation as a largely economic phenomenon. Thanks to modern communications technology, financial transactions have become almost instantaneous, with vast sums of money being moved from New York to Beijing to London at the click of a mouse. Trade liberalisation has produced global markets, in which a few global brands have become ubiquitous, to be found wherever one travels. It has also provoked resistance, of which the 'Occupy' movement is the most recent example. Thanks to modern communication technology, resistance too has a global character. Technology has speeded things up, distances have been contracted. The consequences extend beyond the realms of finance and the economy. Journeys that once only a few people could undertake, and that took days or weeks, are now made by thousands in a matter of hours. The growing scale of population movement, both between countries and from rural areas to cities, has created new challenges for health systems, both quantitatively and qualitatively. In many developing countries economic growth has been highly unequal, with new industrial activity often concentrated on the fringes of huge cities, adjoining impoverished areas that lack decent sanitation, air quality or housing. Such areas 'typically combine the traditional environmental health problems of poverty, particularly respiratory and enteric infections, with those of poor quality housing and unregulated industrialization. Residents are therefore often at risk from diseases and injuries associated with poor sanitation, unsafe drinking water, dangerous roads, polluted air, indoor air pollution and toxic wastes' (McMichael 2000).

The consequences of globalisation extend to the cultural realm too. Cultural products such as pop music and Hollywood movies are to be found almost everywhere, and their stars are now global icons. Images—of war, protest, and disaster—are available to people on the other side of the world at the same time as (or perhaps sooner than) those nearby.

The complex and multifaceted character of globalisation has attracted increasing attention from anthropologists. A key concept in much anthropological writing is that of 'flows' (Inda and Rosaldo 2008). In today's globalised world capital, goods, people, and ideas all travel around the globe with great ease, but they don't do so in identical ways or along the same routes. Political agreements or arrangements facilitate certain kinds of flows (for example flows of capital and products, the unrestricted flow of which is facilitated by international agreements). On the other hand, other flows (such as of migrants) are constrained (by immigration laws and the International Health Regulations referred to in Chapter 1). Nothing flows freely. All flows are structured by material practices (infrastructures, the availability of air links or roads) and by the regulatory practices of governments (opening or closing borders, limiting internet access, encouraging or discouraging foreign investment). Not only do goods, ideas, and people 'flow' in different ways and in different directions, but some localities are far more interconnected than others. Even today there are regions in which the consequences of globalisation may be hard to detect.

A second key notion in the anthropology of globalisation is that of 're-interpretation'. As a product, an image or a practice is transferred from one culture to another, its meaning and significance become fluid, subjected to re-interpretation. This interpretation can have all kinds of consequences. Sometimes two ways of understanding conflict and clashes between cultures result. A currently salient example concerns the all-covering clothing worn by some Muslim women, which some western politicians wish to ban. Sometimes an imported cultural form or practice may be adopted with enthusiasm, for example 'world music' or the 'ethnic' restaurants found in all major cities. As these examples suggest, global flows cannot be understood solely in terms of western 'colonisation', as antiglobalist protests sometimes assume. Flows are more complex and multidirectional. The important point, to be stressed here, is that imported goods, ideas, and practices are subjected to processes of re-interpretation that may lead to adaptation, condemnation or resistance on the part of the receiving community.

An example will enable us to see how these anthropological concepts can be useful in understanding the way immunisation programmes work.

Combatting diarrhoea—rotavirus vaccine

Diarrhoea is the second most common cause of death among children under 5 years of age worldwide (pneumonia being the first). Some 16% of deaths among children aged less than 5 years are a result of diarrheal disease: a loss of about 1.5 million lives annually, more than 80% of them in Africa and South Asia (UNICEF/WHO 2009). The major preventive strategies were laid out decades ago. They correspond more or less to GOBI, emphasised from the mid-1980s onwards. Improved water quality and sanitation, improved nutrition (including the promotion of breastfeeding), better personal and domestic hygiene, and more widespread immunisation would vastly reduce the incidence of diarrhoeal disease. WHO estimates that 88% of deaths from diarrhoea worldwide are the result of unsafe water, inadequate sanitation, and poor hygiene, and that improved water quality and treatment of household water can reduce diarrhoea incidence by as much as 47% (UNICEF/WHO 2009, pp. 11–12).

ORT is the most important treatment, and various anthropological studies of its use, and barriers to its use, have been conducted (e.g. Langsten and Hill 1995). It was quickly recognised that improvements in these aspects of personal and community life, or the acceptability of technologies like ORT, depends on the compatibility of recommended practices with local norms and beliefs. As a result, from the 1980s onwards, numerous studies of local understandings of diarrhoea and its treatment have been conducted in many parts of the world. For example, a study in a rural area of KwaZulu/Natal (South Africa) found that villagers distinguished 11 different types of childhood diarrhoea, each with specific symptoms and characteristics (Kauchali et al. 2004). The researchers classified them as 'diarrhoea of natural causation' (often seen as a normal consequence of physical development such as teething, and not usually felt to need treatment), 'diarrhoea of supernatural causation' (the most commonly reported, typically associated with the breaking of social taboos, and fatal unless ritual healing is practiced), and 'diarrhoea caused by "germs" or diet' (for which ORT is commonly sought). A study in a rural area of Nicaragua found that mothers distinguished nine types of diarrhoea, having distinctive aetiologies ranging from lack of hygiene, certain types of food, worms and parasites, to 'sol de vista' (evil eye) and 'diarrhoea of the sun' (caused by heat) (Davey Smith et al. 1993). Many mothers changed the feeding of their infants when they showed symptoms of diarrhoea, for example some stopped giving their child milk or they gave it rice water. The authors conclude that 'Directly rejecting the mothers' beliefs about diarrhoea, which is what generally occurs in health centres, is not proving to be a fruitful strategy.' The consequences of these differences between lay diarrhoea typologies and those underpinning biomedical thinking and practice are not readily predictable in advance: they may lead to adaptation of prescribed practices and treatments, or they may lead to their rejection.

Improved sanitary measures, breastfeeding, and ORT have considerably reduced overall death from diarrheal disease. This is true of diarrhoea caused by bacteria or parasites, but not by that caused by viruses. Today rotavirus is the major cause of severe gastroenteritis (Bresee et al. 2005; Glass et al. 2005; Bines 2006). Infection occurs most commonly among children aged 6–24 months, with virtually all children (in developed as well as developing countries) infected during their first years of life. In developed countries death from rotavirus infection is rare, although hospitalisation is not. For example, it was estimated that in the USA 1 in 72 children were hospitalised due to a rotavirus infection, and 1 in 19 required medical care before the age of 5. Somewhere between 25 and 55% of hospitalisations for diarrhoea among children under 5 are due to rotavirus infection (Bresee et al. 2005, p. 947). In developing countries rotavirus infections are far more serious than in developed countries. A recent estimate of the number of child deaths associated with rotavirus is 527,000 annually, of which more than 100,000 were in India and 50,000 in Nigeria (Parashar et al. 2009). In the poorest countries approximately one child in 100–200 dies of rotavirus disease by the age of 5. The general opinion is that improved hygienic measures are unlikely to lead to corresponding declines in rotavirus burden.

The virus responsible for rotavirus was identified in 1973. In the early 1980s it was established that first infection, when not fatal, induces immunity to re-infection. This was one reason why it seemed worth trying to develop a vaccine, and attempts to do so began soon after discovery of the virus. The virus is known to consist of a number of different strains, and the first vaccine to be licensed in the world, Wyeth's RotaShield, contained four of them. RotaShield was extensively tested, and trials showed that it conferred 50–60% protection against all cases of rotavirus diarrhoea and 70–100% protection against severe disease. It was licensed by the FDA in 1998, and recommended for routine immunisation of children in three oral doses (at 2, 4, and 6 months). Uptake in the USA was rapid, and within the course of 9 months some 600,000 infants (or approximately 17% of the birth cohort) received the vaccine. However, by July 1999 15 cases of intussusception, a rare but potentially fatal blockage of the intestine, were reported to the US adverse events reporting system (VAERS). Further cases in vaccine recipients were reported thereafter, and a causal link between intussusception and the vaccine seemed probable. Although estimates of the risk of this severe adverse event varied widely, in October 1999 the US Advisory Committee on Immunization Practices and the CDC withdrew their recommendation for RotaShield and the manufacturer voluntarily withdrew it from the market. There was some criticism of this decision. Critics argued that it deprived children in the developing world, for whom rotavirus infection presents a far greater risk than in the USA, of a potentially life-saving innovation (Weijer 2000).

The search for a vaccine continued, and both WHO and GAVI viewed development of safe and effective rotavirus vaccines as a priority. By 2005 both GSK's Rotarix and Merck's RotaTeq vaccines were, or were about to be, licensed. It was understood that the protective efficacy of these vaccines, and the ways in which they should best be used, would differ from place to place. The epidemiology of rotavirus infection was known to differ between developed countries with typically temperate climates and developing countries with (often) tropical ones. 'Differences in age of first infection, strain distribution, seasonality and risk of mortality can affect decisions about vaccine composition, schedule, dose and priority' (Bresee et al. 2005). Both Rotarix and RotaTeq were tested in Europe, North America, and extensively in Latin America. Trials in Mexico, Brazil, and Venezuela showed Rotarix to be 86%

effective against severe rotavirus disease. No significant adverse events were identified. In 2004 Mexico and the Dominican Republic were the first countries to license Rotarix (Bresee et al. 2005).

Although the vaccines were available, and appeared to be effective in the places they had been tested, a number of questions remained before they could become part of the routine immunisation of children worldwide. Would they work in poor areas of Africa and Asia where they were most needed? Since there was often little data on the extent of infection, would countries be interested? Will parents accept a vaccine that protects only against this single cause of childhood diarrhoea? Are they safe? Post-licensure surveillance of hundreds of thousands of children would be needed to ensure that the risk of intussusception was acceptably low. Moreover, depending on the likelihood of infection being fatal, risks and benefits would differ substantially from country to country. What would the vaccines cost and how would they be paid for? Would it be sufficient to rely on the two multinational manufacturers? A problem in this regard was that China, India, and Indonesia, in each of which rotavirus infection was a significant source of infant mortality, relied largely on domestic producers. Neither Merck nor GSK had much penetration into the public sector markets of these countries. In 2006 an application was submitted to GAVI for support for rotavirus introduction in GAVI-eligible countries. The principal applicant was the Rotavirus Vaccine Program of the Seattle-based NGO PATH established in 2003, in collaboration with WHO and CDC.

In 2007 WHO recommended inclusion of rotavirus vaccine in the national immunisation programmes of countries in which a health benefit had been proven in trials, that is, in the Americas and Europe. Recommendations regarding Africa and Asia would have to await the results of trials being carried out there. In 2009 the WHO's Strategic Advisory Group of Experts on Immunisation (generally known by the acronym SAGE) examined their results. SAGE reviewed studies of Rotarix that had been carried out in Malawi and South Africa (completed in July 2008), as well as post-licensure monitoring from Nicaragua, the USA (RotaTeq), and El Salvador (Rotarix) (World Health Organization 2009c).

In the African Rotarix trials, the vaccine had been given alongside the other EPI vaccines, including to HIV-positive infants. The pooled result against severe rotavirus gastroenteritis was 61.25% efficacy (higher in South Africa than in Malawi) and against gastroenteritis from any cause was 30.2%. A study in Nicaragua, one year after introduction of RotaTeq, showed efficacy of 52–63% against severe rotavirus gastroenteritis and 73–86% against very severe gastroenteritis. A study in neighbouring El Salvador, where Rotarix had been introduced, found 74 and 88%. Breastfeeding did not affect the degree of protection afforded.

Based on available data, SAGE recommended that either Rotarix or RotaTeq be given whilst the child is aged 6–15 weeks: two doses could be given together with the first and second DTP shot (World Health Organization 2009a). Adopting the advice of SAGE, WHO agreed that 'rotavirus vaccines are an important measure that can be used to reduce severe rotavirus-associated diarrhoea and child mortality'. It also pointed out that use of the vaccine should be part of a comprehensive strategy to control diarrhoeal diseases, so that its use should be coordinated with other interventions aimed at preventing and treating diarrhoea in children. These include improvement of hygiene and sanitation, use of ORT, and zinc supplementation (World Health Organization 2009c).

It would also be important to ensure that healthcare workers and the general public were accurately and completely informed. Parents and healthcare providers would have to understand that rotavirus infection is the cause of some but not all diarrhoea. A child could be vaccinated and still contract diarrhoea from some other cause.

As trial data came in from more and more regions, it was beginning to seem that the highest protective efficacy of the vaccines was in the countries with the lowest child mortality rates, that is, the measured efficacy was higher in Latin American countries than in African countries. In December 2009 WHO recommended that rotavirus vaccine should be included in all national immunisation programmes. In countries where diarrhoeal deaths account for 10% or more of under-5 mortality, its inclusion was 'strongly recommended'.

In the Americas, where the vaccines had been tried out early on, PAHO analysed experience in the region up till late 2010 (de Oliviera et al. 2011). The study draws on a number of sources, notably the annual immunisation reports that PAHO Member States submit using a standardised PAHO-WHO/UNICEF Joint Reporting Form on Immunization. The authors had access to data on coverage rates (defined as the number of vaccine doses administered divided by the number of children under 1 year), supply failures, and financial information (such as the share of the total cost of the national immunisation programme borne by the government). Data on vaccine safety came from a regional network established for adverse event reporting. A 'sentinel hospital surveillance network', in which hospitals provide monthly reports on rotavirus-related hospital admissions, had been established in 2004. Further information came from the Revolving Fund, the bulk vaccine purchase mechanism that PAHO had established in 1979. Moreover, in 2009 a post-introduction evaluation (PIE study) of the effects of the introduction of rotavirus in Ecuador's immunisation programme had been carried out in collaboration with the Ecuadorian Ministry of

Health and the CDC. Rotavirus vaccine introduction in Ecuador had been particularly successful because disease burden had been established prior to the decision to introduce the vaccine, introduction had been carefully planned, guidelines on vaccine use had been produced and disseminated, and healthcare workers had been trained with specially prepared videos and other material.

Reviewing data from a variety of sources, De Oliviera and colleagues found that by May 2010 15 PAHO member states (42%) had introduced rotavirus vaccine, 6 of them having done so in 2006 (thus the same year the vaccines were licensed in the USA and Europe). Four of the six GAVI-eligible countries in the region (at that time those with a 1999 per capita income of < US$1000) had purchased the vaccine with GAVI support, others had used government funds and the PAHO Revolving Fund. Rotavirus had been introduced much faster than other new vaccines, such as hepatitis B. All except two of the countries used Rotarix in a two-dose schedule, simultaneously with other routine antigens. However, in all of the countries rotavirus coverage was lower than these other antigens. 'In countries with less than 50% rotavirus coverage for children with a vaccine effectiveness of approximately 70% against severe diarrhoea gastroenteritis, the intervention would have a limited effect' (De Oliviera et al. 2011). Why is rotavirus coverage lower than coverage of the other EPI vaccines? A number of possible reasons are discussed, including the age restriction for rotavirus immunisation (due to risk of intussusception) and logistical problems. But these authors have nothing to say about what ethnographic studies had shown. There is no reference to the finding that in some communities diarrhoea was categorised in quite different ways, some forms of which might be seen as the result of supernatural causes or as a normal aspect of child development.

In 2009 UNICEF and WHO set out a seven-point plan for tackling diarrhoea mortality and morbidity (UNICEF/WHO 2009). Two of the seven points refer to treatments (ORT above all, and now zinc treatment, which has been shown to reduce severity and duration). Five of them refer to preventive measures such as improved water supplies and sanitation, breastfeeding, and rotavirus immunisation. To what extent current prioritisation of rotavirus vaccine introduction is affecting attention to these other aspects of diarrhoea control is not clear (Esser and Bench 2011). What is clear is that the global market for rotavirus vaccines is growing rapidly. By 2009 it had reached almost US$1 billion. New sources of production are emerging. In China, India, and Indonesia—large countries that rely largely on domestic vaccine producers—rotavirus vaccines are being developed. In China the Lanzhou Institute of Biological Products LLR vaccine was licensed in China as early as 2000 (although not exported). In June 2011 an Indian biotechnology company, Bharat Biotech, announced that its

Rotavac vaccine was being tested in Phase III clinical trials, with licensing expected in 2014. The price of fully immunising a child would then be US$3, compared to US$5 or US$7.50 at present. In addition, the BMGF-supported Program of Appropriate Technology for Health (PATH) is working to assist local vaccine manufacturers in Brazil, India, and China to develop rotavirus vaccines (World Health Organization 2011b).

Within 5 or 6 years rotavirus vaccines had moved from the laboratories of the multinational pharmaceutical companies who were developing them to the bodies of children worldwide. This could be seen simply as a case of successful market expansion. But there is another, more anthropological perspective, and anthropological concepts such as 'flow' and 'interpretation' may give us some insights into this process.

We can distinguish three analytic steps. Who and what is involved? Where and how do they encounter each other? What goes on at these encounters?

Diffusion (or 'flow') of the vaccine involved numerous participants. Some international organisations played important roles. Both WHO and GAVI had stated that development of a rotavirus vaccine was a public health priority, and this may have acted as an incentive to the pharmaceutical industry. WHO, acting on the advice of its expert advisory group (SAGE), issued recommendations regarding introduction of the vaccine to national immunisation programmes. In the Americas PAHO went further, through establishment of a regional surveillance system for reporting of adverse events, through supporting national governments in purchasing vaccine supplies through its Revolving Fund, and through studies of national experiences. GAVI played an important role in providing grants for vaccine purchase to the poorest of countries. The CDC and PATH, although not intergovernmental organisations, also played important roles by, for example, applying to GAVI for support of rotavirus purchase.

Clearly national governments also played key roles. Their commitment could not be taken for granted, since there was frequently little data on the burden of rotavirus-related disease. As Glass et al. noted in 2005: 'Despite the availability of simple, sensitive and inexpensive test kits, a diagnosis of rotavirus disease is rarely sought, and it would be hard to introduce a new vaccine against a disease whose local importance is unrecognized' (Glass et al. 2005). Similarly, Cunliffe and Nakagomi write that 'Despite international recognition that rotavirus gastro-enteritis is an important cause of death in children, at country level rotavirus has not been viewed as a pathogen of major importance' (Cunliffe and Nakagomi 2007). They stress the importance of collecting country-specific data, both in demonstrating the local efficacy of the vaccine and in making rotavirus diarrhoea a clearer public health priority. Some countries (including El Salvador, Malawi, and Nicaragua) nevertheless facilitated the establishment of clinical trials of candidate vaccines. The vaccine had to be licensed by national regulatory authorities and then, perhaps, the decision taken to introduce it to the national immunisation programme. Ideally, this involved careful preparation (expansion of the cold chain, training health workers, arranging distribution of the new vaccine), as was done in Ecuador. Arrangements for reporting to donors on changes in disease incidence vaccine uptake would almost certainly be required. SAGE had recommended that rotavirus vaccination programmes be coordinated with other interventions to prevent and treat childhood diarrheal diseases, such as improvement of hygiene and sanitation, use of ORT, and zinc supplementation. If this was to be done, it too would have to be planned by governments.

Health workers, whether operating from child health centres or from mobile vaccination units, are the ones who have to do the immunising. If use of the vaccine is indeed to be coordinated with other antidiarrheal measures, then it would be the health workers who would have to educate the mothers in the importance of these measures, provide zinc supplements, and so on.

Finally, but crucially, mothers have to be able and willing to bring their infants to be vaccinated. 'Able' because, as research has shown, many features of the organisation of immunisation programmes may create significant constraints. Such features include accessibility of the vaccination centre and the likelihood that vaccine will in fact be available. Willingness of mothers to bring their infants to be vaccinated against rotavirus will also be influenced by their understanding of what precisely they are being offered, by the attitude of staff, and by other factors. Would parents accept a vaccine for only one cause of childhood diarrhoea? (As Glass et al. put it: 'A nagging question remains as to whether mothers might feel cheated or misled if their child received a rotavirus vaccine but still developed diarrhoea, albeit of a different aetiology. For example, a mother in Bangladesh would hardly recognize the effects of the vaccine because her child might experience 20–30 episodes of diarrhoea during the first 5 years of life, only 1 of which is due to rotavirus' (Glass et al. 2005, p. S165).) And here again local understandings and categorisations of diarrheal disease become relevant.

The concepts of 'chains' and 'interfaces'

This example of rotavirus vaccine is illustrative of the processes of diffusion, or flow, on which a successful vaccination programme depends. Vaccines flow from sites of global (although perhaps increasingly regional) production in the first place to national health authorities. But vaccines themselves are not all that is required. Information flows also play a crucial role. On the basis of advice from SAGE, WHO issues recommendations for the use of the vaccines: which countries should use them, who should receive them, at what age they should be administered, and in how many doses. Flows of financial resources may also be critical. Many poor countries that have introduced rotavirus vaccination have done so with the aid of funds from the GAVI Alliance. Thereafter, national health authorities distribute materials, instructions, resources, and personnel to the regional and community levels. This takes place through a mix of infra-structural and policy mechanisms. A cold chain must be in place, instructions issued. Health workers, armed with suitable materials, with instructions and reporting forms, then engage with the communities for which they are respon-sible, and with the mothers and the children living there. Anthropologists Leach and Fairhead's statement that 'at the needle point the most global meets the most personal of worlds' seems apt indeed (Leach and Fairhead 2007, p. 2).

It is helpful to think of this 'vaccination chain' in terms of a series of distinctive levels—the global, national, local, and personal. In reality, this is a simplification, and the 'levels' are not as clearly distinguished, or as stable, as this suggests. 'The global', for example, is not a permanent configuration of institutions with fixed mandates and ways of working. In Chapter 1 we referred to the emergence of conflicting perspectives on primary and selective primary health care held by WHO and UNICEF that influenced development of EPI. Reconfigurations, changes in the configuration of global institutions concerned with public health policy, the struggle for influence, resources and leadership continue (as discussed further in Chapter 3). In large countries like India the regional level plays an important role: the responsibilities of the individual states are much more com-plex than the simple implementation of central government policy. On the other hand, in small countries such as Malawi the regional level may be little more than a node in the distribution system. Moreover, the levels interpenetrate each other in ways that vary from place to place and over time. For example, national experts may sit on WHO advisory panels, whilst WHO may be represented within the country by a national office. We return to this point below. Within the country also similar processes of interpenetration are at play. National vaccine policies are often powerfully shaped by popular anxieties: communities demanding a vaccine or, by contrast, responding to rumours of its risks and refusing it. The state is present in the local community, symbolically and materially, in a host of ways. The public health facilities on which families depend for much of their treatment, care, and advice in a sense also represent the state. How receptive to a vaccination message mothers might be might well reflect more general satisfaction with the service provided. But it might also reflect quite different sentiments of a general social or political nature. Political cleavages or discontents, just as much as short-age of resources or culturally insensitive staff, can influence how mothers respond to vaccination advice (Roalkvam and Sandberg 2010). To assume we can think about these levels independently is a simplification, but it is a useful one.

How and where do these levels intersect: the global with the national, the national with the local, and so on? If observers were to describe these many different interfaces on the basis of what they saw, their descriptions would seem to have little in common. We would be given descriptions of events ranging from the annual WHA in Geneva to the arrival of a mobile vaccination team in an African village. What they have in common is that each event has an ostensible purpose that is sufficiently acknowledged to make attendance seem worthwhile. Participants arrive with different sets of assumptions, values, intentions, and interests, and in interacting they will seek consensus, accommodation, to get out what they came for at an acceptable price, or whatever it may be. What can we say about these interfaces? First, although over time they may slowly change, they are relatively stable sites at which interactions occur over and again. For example, the interfaces between health workers and health seekers, or a national public health bureaucracy and the regional WHO representative, persist in an organised way over time. There are generally well-established rules, sanctions, procedures, and ways of handling conflicting interests and perceptions.

Second, although interface interactions presuppose some degree of agreement (for example regarding rules and procedures) they frequently generate tensions or conflict due to unequal power relations, or conflicting loyalties or commitments. For example, a lay health worker, often a member of a local community working for an immunisation programme in that community, may face conflicting values or expectations. She must respond to the demands of her own community as well as to the expectations of the health systems managers to whom she is responsible (for examples of how health workers in India are affected by these tensions see Sheikh and George 2010). She must constantly negotiate her position between these two domains. When mothers in rural north India meet with state health workers they negotiate immunisation practice with reference to their own personal network (cf. Gupta 1995). With reference to India, Corbridge et al. (2005) argue that the success and roll out of all contemporary new state programmes is heavily dependent on how these positions are negotiated both by governmental workers and community members. The dynamics of contradiction, ambivalence, and loyalties at any interface needs to be empirically established rather than assumed (Nordfeldt and Roalkvam 2010).

In other words interfaces are characterised by on the one hand a certain stability with established rules and procedures, and on the other by the juxtaposition of distinctive and potentially conflicting sets of values, beliefs, rationalities, and intentions (Long 1989, 2001). The analytic value of the concept is that it will help us make comparisons both along the 'vaccine chain' in any one country and between countries. Nevertheless, in doing so we will have to bear in mind that each specific instance must be situated in relation to broader domains of culture, knowledge, and power, which differ from country to country. What participants bring to the interaction significantly influences what goes on there.

'Interface work'—compliance or re-interpretation?

The next step in our argument involves addressing the question 'What goes on at these interfaces?' In line with anthropological writing, we referred to it as a process of 're-interpretation'. How does an anthropological perspective such as we are suggesting actually help, and is re-interpretation the right term for what appears to be going on?

As we saw in the previous chapter, technologies, targets, and the global perspective have become increasingly central to international health policy. These are the dimensions against which national 'performance' is judged. It is taken for granted that new vaccines recommended by WHO should be introduced rapidly to national immunisation schedules. Failure to be compliant is then seen as deviant behaviour, in need of explanation. Various studies have sought to distinguish between, and compare, rapid- and late-adopting countries. Detailed studies of national decision-making processes, however, tend to show that decisions emerge from a complex interplay of actors and arguments (e.g. Munira and Fritzen 2007).

Consider the vaccine against human papilloma virus (HPV). Since 2009 WHO has recommended routine administration of HPV vaccines to preadolescent girls in countries where cervical cancer prevention is recognised as a public health priority and where vaccine introduction is programmatically and financially feasible. Since April 2012 GAVI-eligible countries have been able to apply for support for HPV introduction. Many rich industrialised countries introduced HPV vaccine some years earlier. Haas and colleagues looked at what had happened in seven countries, each of which introduced it in 2006 (Haas et al. 2009). Public debate proceeded in parallel with, or subsequent to, the decision to subsidise vaccination from public funds. The nature of the policy debate differed from country to country. In some countries the manufacturers were very visible (and concern at their influence on politicians may have stimulated resistance to the programmes); in other countries they were not. Medical associations and consumer advocacy groups played important, but varied, roles. Thus in Canada, New Zealand, Australia and the USA most medical and public health agencies and societies supported a voluntary subsidised programme. In both Canada and New Zealand women's health advocacy organisations either opposed the programme or expressed concerns about the speed of introduction and the lack of knowledge regarding long-term effects. In the USA and Canada moral issues, relating to possible encouragement of earlier sexual activity, were raised by religious and conservative groups. The controversy that has surrounded HPV vaccine, especially in North America, has attracted a lot of attention from anthropologists and sociologists (e.g. see Wailoo et al. 2010).

Formally speaking, Ministries of Health play key roles in deciding on the introduction of new vaccines. But Ministries of Health are subject to all kinds of influences, both from 'above' (WHO, the pharmaceutical industry) and from 'below' (communities, advocacy groups, professions). And although disease burden is likely to be cited in justification of the decision to introduce a new vaccine, political realities are much more complex. On the one hand, health policy-makers everywhere are under pressure to conform to international guidelines, to standardise immunisation schedules, and rapidly to introduce new vaccines. But they also have to deal with public opinion ('pressure from below'). In some countries far more than in others, political realities mean that health policy-makers must listen carefully to the anxieties and opinions emerging from society. How far this is so depends on the country's political culture. Are civil society groups that advocate on behalf of women's health, or community health, or specific groups of patients well organised? Do they have access to the mass media? Do they have the expertise to contest official claims and data? When civil society organisations possess the legitimacy, the degree of organisation, and the expertise to influence health policy and politics, the politics of new vaccine introduction may be changed dramatically.

India, with its vibrant civil society and a long tradition of political activism, is particularly interesting in this regard. In India the introduction of HPV vaccine has not proceeded in the way global sponsors anticipated. In 2009, with support from the BMGF, and in collaboration with the Indian Council of Medical Research (ICMR) and the state governments, PATH launched a study of HPV vaccine in the states of Andhra Pradesh and Gujarat (Sarojini et al. 2010). The study was described as a 'demonstration project'. In March 2010 a team of women's rights activists visited one of the study sites, interviewing girls who had been vaccinated and health staff, and looking to establish how consent had been obtained, what information had been provided, and what kind of health infrastructure was available to support cancer screening and prevention. They found that many trial participants were from particularly disadvantaged backgrounds and communities, that health infrastructures were 'woefully inadequate', and that large numbers of girls and their parents were unaware that they were part of a research project. The activists concluded that procedures had violated all relevant ethical guidelines. There had been no follow-up of the four deaths believed to have been caused by the vaccination, and apparently the numerous side-effects reported to the team of activists had been neither recorded in the official study nor investigated. The report of this fact-finding mission led to a public outcry, such that in April 2010 the central government health minister announced a halt to all HPV vaccine trials in the country. Sarojini and her colleagues raise a whole range of questions concerning the influence of multi-national pharmaceutical companies, international organisations, and foreign NGOs on the country's health policies and priorities. They question the rationality of introducing a vaccine that is unproven in India, and the cost of which is likely to draw resources from already inadequate screening services. 'The vaccine,' they write, 'cannot be a substitute for comprehensive public health services'. It is the causes of vulnerability, including the absence of health care, that need to be addressed.

Interventions by global institutions may encounter resistance at all levels of Indian society. Kavita Sivaramakrishnan's analysis of the international, national, and regional responses to a suspected outbreak of plague in the city of Surat, in the Indian State of Gujarat, illustrates clearly how and why this might occur (Sivaramakrishnan 2011). In 1994 an outbreak of what appeared to be plague was reported in Surat. The regional government denied that it was plague, arguing that it was pneumonia, and the national government failed to send any notification to WHO (as IHRs required in the case of plague). WHO, engaged in establishing a more active and more central role for itself, wished to investigate. The Indian government was reluctant to allow it to do so, a reluctance which Sivaramakrishnan attributes to the commitment of the Indian state to its own sovereignty and self-reliance. It eventually gave way in the face of attention from national media and pressure from neighbouring countries. When the team of WHO experts did visit the region they found local scientists uncooperative, and their report offered no clear picture of the nature or origins of the disease. Thereafter the Indian government appointed its own committee of inquiry comprising scientists drawn from leading research institutions. This committee confirmed that the outbreak was in fact plague, although the strain of Yersinia Pestis was an unknown one. Since its origins could not be explained, major uncertainties remained. Finally, the state government of Gujarat appointed its own committee of inquiry. Whereas the national committee consisted largely of microbiologists and biochemists, the Gujarat committee also included experts in social medicine, and its report struck a very different tone. Introducing themes of poverty, unplanned industrialisation, and unregulated migration, the Gujarat committee explained the outbreak in terms of urban environmental deterioration and the effects of the industrial policies of the national government. 'Causal explanations for the same event differed widely on the basis of political projects and context, showing that global health crises can reflect several distinct political projects simultaneously' (Sivaramakrishnan 2011, p. 1039). Nevertheless, the author argues, the Surat outbreak was later used as a reference point by WHO in seeking support for a global disease surveillance network and to 'ensure greater cooperation from states in public health governance'.

Countries lacking India's size, economic dynamism, and political traditions only rarely offer such resistance to global pressures to conform. Their Ministries of Health are increasingly responsive to signals from the global level, rather than signals from the local community, from which they have become increasingly disconnected.

Over time, a shift has taken place in the relations between national and international institutions. Interactions in which national governments sought technical help and support for public health (including immunisation) priorities emerging from domestic politics have given way to interactions at which global funds are used to catalyse the implementation of global health policies.

Stepping back a bit in time for a moment helps us get some perspective on these changes. Somewhere between the late 1940s and the 1970s many countries in Africa and Asia gained independence from colonial rule. Their governments began to formulate policies to promote the economic and social welfare of their populations. Institutional structures inherited from the colonial period would have to be adapted or redesigned. In many countries deep scars left by violent struggles for independence had to be healed. Still, in the 1950s and 1960s many Asian and African countries were doing well. They enjoyed considerable rates of economic growth. Starting in the 1980s this began to change, and rates of economic growth began to fall. Why was this? Political economist Alice Amsden has examined the impact of US policy on development, and on institutions such as the World Bank that are there to support it (Amsden 2007). She argues that the USA forced a transformation in the policies and practices of developing countries. Whereas until the 1980s the American government was saying 'do it your way' (so encouraging countries to develop their own institutions, policies, and thinking), from the 1980s onwards it was saying 'do it our way'. Developing countries suffered from the 1980s onwards because they were under pressure to conform to a particular model of trade and economic development. Does something similar hold for public health? Consider the case of Uganda.

At independence from British colonial rule, in 1962, Uganda inherited a health system that prioritised hospital medicine and the needs of the urban population (Okuonzi and Macrae 1995). A series of violent changes of regime, and the repressive government of Idi Amin, resulted in a breakdown of health services. International NGOs filled the gap, although independently and in the absence of any overall coordination. Their emphasis tended to be on vertical programmes, including immunisation, that seemed the most feasible at the time. When the National Resistance Movement came to power in 1986, these vertical programmes were expanded—the hope being that they could provide a platform for developing primary health care. Attempts at developing a new national health policy soon began, but little progress was made. In the absence of a clear health policy framework, initiatives funded and organised from outside the country continued to play a major role: in effect limiting the possibilities of a strategic health services plan. In 1991 a national 10-year health Plan WAS developed, but since the budget required was vastly greater than resources, it prompted a protest on the part of donors. The concern of donors, especially the World Bank, led to the increasing involvement of international advisors in policy-making. In order to ensure that 'appropriate' health policies were formulated, policy-making processes and planning capacity had to be strengthened. In 1992 a 3-year plan 'largely developed by expatriate advisers' was published (Okuonzi and Macrae 1995). In 1992 the World Bank made a new healthcare loan, subject to the condition that user fees were introduced. A study carried out ten years later suggests that the result has been an MoH tightly connected to the global public health community, but disconnected from its own local communities (Jeppsson et al. 2005). The MoH 'is rather part of a system that operates in the respective country as well as in a global "center" rather than a part of an indigenous process' (Jeppsson et al. 2005, p. 318). The autonomy in policy-making the country had briefly enjoyed, which had led to a strategic plan unacceptable to international donors, had gone.

Taken together, these two Ugandan studies help us understand how and why 'what happens' at the global–national interface has changed, and in ways not dissimilar to what Amsden found in the field of economic development. Changing relations between national health policy-making and the global level have been a consequence of an evolution in the structure of the global level, and of the assumptions underpinning the policies of donor institutions. National health authorities have to deal with an increasing variety of global institutions and donor agencies, with distinctive agendas and ways of working. Crucially, institutions like WHO that provide technical support and advice, but little financial support, have come to be dominated by others (such as the World Bank, GAVI, and philanthropic organisations such as the BMGF) that provide essential funds for health projects, but subject to strict conditionalities. And most importantly, it appears that these global institutions increasingly intervene in the processes through which national policies are formulated.

Expatriate advisors played key roles in developing the 1992 Uganda health plan. We know from other studies that this was not something peculiar to Uganda (or indeed to the health field). Jackson studied the work of development agencies in Honduras (Jackson 2005). What he found was a gradual marginalisation of local experts and professionals, their advisory role being taken over by expatriate advisors. He concludes 'Only local agendas linking into the global ones are going to succeed, and only Honduran institutions giving their consent to globalization are likely to prosper' (Jackson 2005, p. 126). Goldman has shown how the World Bank, through training local policy analysts, has been able to shape 'what counts' as environmental knowledge in accordance with its own agenda (Goldman 2005). The result is that in place of responding to the needs of local communities, from which they have become disconnected, Ministries of Health are both pressurised and encouraged to implement global priorities with as little delay as possible.

The tendency in global public health analysis, as we have seen, is to assume compliance (for example in following recommendations for the introduction of a new vaccine) and to try to explain the 'deviant' behaviour of those who fail to comply. Our perspective here is different. In other words, when focusing on what goes on at interfaces, our objective is not to judge the extent to which advice is being followed as we move down the chain. Our perspective requires that we avoid privileging the perspective of one participant or another. The significance of this can be illustrated by reference to writing on 'vaccine refusal': the seemingly growing influence of 'antivaccination movements' in many countries of the global North. Much of what public health experts have to say on this matter takes for granted that parents rejecting vaccination for their child are acting illogically or on the basis of misinformation disseminated (via the internet) by antivaccination organisations. Emphasis is then placed on countering this misinformation. The assumption is that if parents were adequately informed regarding the risks of infectious diseases, and the extent to which these risks can be reduced by vaccination, they would act rationally and differently. By contrast we assume that parents' actions are based on evidence or convictions that make good sense to them, in the light of their own or friends' and neighbours' experiences, however much these differ from clinical or epidemiological understandings. Only after these distinctive understandings, and their roots, have been understood can a culturally appropriate health education strategy be designed. In similar vein George Davey Smith and his colleagues, who studied diarrhoea prevention in Nicaragua, concluded that 'Directly rejecting the mothers' beliefs about diarrhoea, which is what generally occurs in health centres, is not proving to be a fruitful strategy' (Davey Smith 1993). The controversy surrounding the introduction of cervical cancer vaccine, a controversy that public health officials had not anticipated—illustrates the importance of the distinction.

The crucial concept for us, in other words, is not 'compliance', but 're-interpretation'. 'What goes on' at the interfaces are processes of re-interpretation.

Vaccination is not always understood in terms of enhanced protection (whether of the child or of the community) against a specific pathogen. Sometimes mothers think that vaccination will protect a child's health 'in general', rather than prevent a specific disease. Misunderstandings between health workers and mothers may become all the greater when the disease the vaccine is supposed to protect against corresponds only partly, or not at all, with a local illness term. Clashes of meaning such as this are to be found in interactions between health professionals and mothers in the global North as well as in the global South. For example, in both Britain and the USA many parents seem to make a distinction (that medical science denies) between 'natural immunity' and the 'artificial immunity' conferred by immunisation (Leach and Fairhead 2007, p. 52), or they believe that a small child's immune system can be 'overloaded' (Leach and Fairhead 2007, p. 55). It is because vaccination links the intimate sphere of the body to broader social and political spheres that vaccination programmes sometimes provide a focus for social and political disaffections. This is why conspiracy theories are not uncommon in vaccine history. For example, in the 1990s the rumour emerged in the Philippines that tetanus vaccination of adult women was being used for family planning purposes (Streefland et al. 1999; see also Kaler 2009). A more recent example is the following.

As we discussed in Chapter 1, in 1988 the WHA committed WHO to the global eradication of polio by the year 2000. Shortage of financial resources is one reason why the eradication target date has had continuously to be extended, but it is not the only one. Unanticipated outbreaks of the disease, particularly in West Africa and South Asia, have also been a major setback to the campaign. So far as a resurgence of polio infections in West Africa is concerned, events that took place in northern Nigeria, starting in 2003, are often said to have played a significant role (Yahya 2007). In that year, religious leaders in the predominantly Muslim states of northern Nigeria claimed to have discovered that the oral polio vaccine being used had been deliberately contaminated with antifertility drugs and AIDS-inducing agents. Five northern states banned use of the vaccine in their respective areas: a move that attracted considerable critical attention in western media. Obadare has sought to explain these events, and the reasons for northern Nigerian mistrust both of WHO and UNICEF (sponsors of the programme) and of the Federal government, in terms of the legacy of colonialism and the region's post-colonial history (Obadare 2005). 'To sum up, the polio vaccination crisis as a whole provides a paradigm of emergent tensions between the North and the South that are best understood in light of historical relations between the two. . . . it also clearly shows up the deepening immersion of health in the domain of politics, coupled with the increasingly political nature of health issues in the contemporary world' (Obadare 2005, p. 278). The country's internal politics are no less at issue, in particular the ongoing post-independence contestation between the country's main ethnic groups over political power and autonomy. Northern Nigerians mistrusted a Federal government that had recently come under southern domination. Mistrust was fuelled by a sense that it was Federal government policy that had led to the erosion of already inadequate primary health care. As Yahya's research showed, people simply could not understand why this one disease was receiving such (disproportionate) resources, when most people couldn't afford basic medicines to treat even minor ailments.

Trust is crucial: trust in vaccines, trust in the professionals who administer them, trust in the government and the health system under which those professionals work. But it cannot be taken for granted. Like the widespread controversy around HPV vaccine, what happened in Nigeria shows the fragility of this trust. Controversies like these show that vaccination campaigns can provide the opportunity for anxieties and prejudices to be made explicit. The Nigerian polio controversy also shows us that national perceptions of 'global' or 'the nation' have to be understood in context. Inflected by a people's history of engagement with the international order, whether as colonised or coloniser, by struggles for independence, by a history of ethnic conflict or its lack, the beneficence of global (or national) institutions may be doubted. When we wrote earlier of the need to situate specific instances of interfacing 'in relation to broader domains of culture, knowledge, and power', this is part of what we meant. The challenge, then, is to tease out those broader themes in collective memory that are likely to influence the ways in which any modification to an immunisation programme will be interpreted.

The analytical framework

How does the perspective outlined here help us understand the complex process by which vaccines reach the bodies of children? Where does it direct our attention and what questions does it encourage us to ask? We have introduced the concept of 'flows', central to much anthropological writing on global phenomena. It suggests that we need to examine the flows of things, ideas, and information, as well as differences between and disruptions to these flows. What is it that 'flows' through the vaccine system? The vaccine, which has to be distributed through a carefully maintained cold chain, literally does 'flow'. Some disappears along the way, as we will see. Information flows too, although differently. WHO and its regional offices issue recommendations and disseminate information of the kind that government decision-makers might find important or persuasive, and often in a quantitative form, for example recommending introduction of the rotavirus vaccine, 'In Africa and Asia alone, a vaccine with approximately 60% efficacy has the potential to save more than 1.5 million lives in the period from 2010 to 2025' (World Health Organization 2009b). Information, however, flows in both directions, since countries are expected to submit data on coverage and morbidity to WHO, health centres to national authorities, health workers to their supervisors. And money flows too, perhaps via an international organisation (for example a GAVI grant, or through the PAHO Revolving Fund).

We have emphasised the importance of interfaces as especially deserving of research attention. But instead of regarding these as sites at which instructions flowing down from above are followed more or less exactly, we regard them as sites of re-interpretation. From an anthropological perspective one has to attend to the ways in which technologies, practices, ideas or images (so including vaccines and assumptions regarding their use) may change meanings as they travel from one culture, or one society, to another. That is to say, we have to try to understand how such things are understood in terms of the interests to which a national government has to respond or the concepts meaningful in the adopting culture. How does a Zulu mother, who distinguishes 11 different kinds of diarrhoea—of which the most common is that due to supernatural causes—understand a measure designed to protect her child against rotavirus? Whether she ultimately decides for or against vaccination, and on whatever grounds, her first step is surely to make sense of what it is that she is being invited, advised or pressured to have done to her child.

Fundamental to the analysis presented here is the attempt to avoid privileging the perspective of any participant in the vaccination chain and (following from this) to avoid any kind of moral condemnation or blame. What follows from this starting point is a need to analyse 'positive' decisions (vaccine adoption or acceptance) and 'negative' decisions (non-adoption or vaccine rejection) in the same way. This applies whether we are looking at the introduction (or non-introduction) of a new vaccine, or acceptance or rejection by an individual mother. In this we thus depart from most writing from a public health perspective. Second, 'numbers' (for example measures of vaccine coverage) have to be understood as socially constructed in the light of pressures and expectations with which actors are confronted, as well as the uses to which such numbers will be put. Third, in examining what goes on at the various interfaces identified we must (a) situate the distinctive interfaces in relation to the broader domains of knowledge and power in which they are embedded and (b) try to make explicit the knowledge, experience, and expectations that each participant brings to the interaction, as well as the unfolding over time of relationships between them. Fourth, we will be particularly sensitive to discontinuities in understandings of what vaccines are and how they work, and the kind of evidence or beliefs that people bring in support of their views.

A principal implication is that when it seems that policy measures (such as immunisation) that from a public health point of view are vital are nevertheless resisted, the next step is to try to understand the nature of—or the grounds for—that resistance. To seek a solution that respects deeply held concerns or beliefs even where these seem irrational from a medical point of view often leads in unfamiliar directions.

The resistance of northern Nigerian Muslims to the polio campaign showed a loss of trust in the vaccine and in the agencies (national and international) that provided the vaccine and supported the campaign. Northern Nigerians had reasons for doubting that these agencies had their best interests at heart, and the polio vaccine came to symbolise their disaffection. When the Federal Nigerian government claimed to have established scientifically that the vaccine was safe, their findings lacked legitimacy. In this context the following is worthy of note. In considering the introduction of a new vaccine to their well-functioning national immunisation programmes, European countries have tended (at least until recently) to give serious attention to implications for popular trust in the immunisation programme as a whole. In recommending the introduction of new vaccines in poor countries, however, it seems that the effectiveness of the vaccine alone is to be determinant.

Legitimacy and trust are key concepts here. The legitimacy of decisions taken by politicians and their public health advisors may be called into question on a variety of grounds: that the political elite is not representative of the country's ethnic or regional structure, that it is compromised by personal interests, that people have a fundamental right to participate in decisions concerning their health and well-being. A loss of trust in a particular vaccine, perhaps based on rumour, or on appeals to gaps in the evidence for its effectiveness, or on claims that evidence has been biased by commercial interests (as happened in the wake of the recent panic over H1N1 influenza), or in the institutions supporting the immunisation programme can have similar consequences. Where legitimacy or trust break down, where local communities or advocacy organisations debate aspects of vaccination that matter to them in their own terms and insist on being heard, the work of interpretation becomes integral to the decision-making process.

Taking for granted that public health is a necessarily global responsibility, the tendency is to view decision-making unidirectionally. National authorities should act in accordance with priorities and objectives set at the global level, communities with those of the national government. Performance is then assessed on this basis. Social scientists who have explored the working of immunisation programmes at the community level not uncommonly see things differently. Thus Das et al., reviewing the results of a series of studies carried out in India in the 1990s, emphasise the importance of building capabilities and competences at the community level if immunisation (and other health services) are to be used effectively (Das et al. 2000). That these approaches lead in different directions is well illustrated by the example of surveillance. No-one questions the importance of a well-functioning surveillance system. Epidemiological surveillance allows decision-makers to respond to changing circumstances: to the emergence of a local disease outbreak for example, to the emergence of resistance, or to a shift in the age-distribution of incidence. Indeed, the new IHRs are designed in part to strengthen national (and more particularly international) disease surveillance. How this is to be accomplished is problematic, given the possible reluctance of national governments to acknowledge disease outbreaks, but also given limited health service and laboratory testing facilities. A recent paper has contrasted the surveillance systems operating in a number of countries (Calain 2006a). In Laos, the author found a variety of systems operating in parallel with that of the MoH, uncoordinated, each with its own approach and each funded by a different global programme or international donor. In Cambodia, by contrast, he found a system in which village health volunteers were trained to identify and report on certain diseases, syndromes, and clusters of events. An evaluation attributed the success of this system to its simplicity and its decentralised management. In South India too, the well-known vaccinologist T. Jacob John had established a low-budget bottom-up approach that had effectively identified emerging disease outbreaks. The Cambodian and South Indian experiments are 'far away from the gravitational forces of major donor agencies' (Calain 2006a). Calain is concerned that implementing the global surveillance agenda is likely more to disrupt than to benefit the fragile health systems of poor countries.

What difference could it make?

It is not merely for the sake of intellectual challenge that we try to replace elements in the conceptual scheme dominating international health with concepts taken from the social sciences. Our concern is to establish how vaccines, as powerful tools of public health, can best be deployed in the interests of children's health and well-being. What kind of a difference might the change of perspective we advocate make in practice?

What does a high level of vaccine coverage actually tell us? Anthropologist Mark Nichter has argued that high vaccine coverage could be the result of 'active demand' for the vaccine or of its 'passive acceptance' (Nichter 1995). By 'active demand' he means 'adherence to vaccination programs by an informed public which perceives the benefits of and need for specific vaccinations'. Passive acceptance, on the other hand, means compliance: a public which 'yields to the recommendations and social pressure, if not prodding, of health workers and community leaders'. If vaccination programmes are to be sustainable then, according to Nichter, enhancement of 'community demand', not increased coverage rate, should be the goal. The tendency has been to assume that once high coverage had been achieved people would soon see the benefits: a conclusion that is not supported by community-level studies. Reviewing numerous studies carried out in South and South-East Asia, Nichter's conclusion is that vaccinations are generally 'accepted passively as a result of interactions with health care providers and because compliance is demanded by those in positions of power. Demand is often low, even among populations having impressive immunization rates.' (Nichter 1995, p. 625). Arguing along similar lines, Streefland et al. have shown how passive vaccine acceptance may result from the structure of a local community. 'Prevailing forms of social inequality may help people adhere to the vaccination rules, since the socially weak (landless peasants, young mothers) will easily conform if the village elite sets the rules' (Streefland et al. 1999, p. 1708). Drawing on previous research in Indonesia, they point out how health service administrations may work with and through the local village elite, leading the majority of poor villagers to feel they have to conform.

On the basis of their studies in India, Das et al. make a similar argument. It is not correct, they argue, to make a clear distinction between communities that want the vaccine and those that reject it because of resistance shaped by local beliefs. High and low coverage are the result of the interplay of a variety of factors: ecological features (physical isolation, poor infrastructure making travel difficult) and social features (isolation of elements within a community due to hierarchy based on caste or ethnicity). There are important implications both for research and for the objectives that policy should address. Thus, they argue for a shift in the focus of epidemiological research from the individual or the household to the community as a whole. 'Our studies show that it is not literacy at the household level that affects demand for vaccination. . . . However there is a sharp difference in demand for and acceptance of vaccination between communities which have a thin layer of educated women versus those which may have literate ones but not educated ones in the community'. (Das et al. 2000, p. 628). Crucial is the existence in the community of a critical number of educated women.

A shift in emphasis from coverage rates to community demand implies a shift in the focus of research away from predictors of individual demand and towards characteristics of communities. Thus Nichter argues that researchers should switch their attention to the values and beliefs largely shared in the communities in which individuals live. Cultural factors, including understandings of disease and protection, become crucial in such an analysis. For example, do people perceive the benefits of vaccination as preventing a specific illness or as simply being good for the child's health? Is a vaccine perceived as preventing a specific disease or as offering a child a more general protection (which would put it on a par with other kinds of talismans)? How can the working of vaccines be explained to people who don't believe in diseases having specific distinct causes? If people believe that immunisation confers general protection on their child, they may reasonably feel that one or two are sufficient: it matters little which. Similar reasoning leads Streefland et al. to the notion of 'local vaccination cultures'. They define the term as follows: 'Shared notions emerge when relatives or neighbours exchange accounts of their vaccination experiences . . . which then colour their subsequent experiences. Together with prevailing beliefs about disease aetiology, ideas about the potency and efficacy of modern medicine, and views on the need for preventive health measures, these shared notions may be called local vaccination cultures' (Streefland et al. 1999, p. 1707).

Das et al. interpret their findings as showing 'the importance of building social capital in the community for effective utilization of the social services offered by the state.' Their community level studies show that 'though conceived as a technocratic solution towards reducing morbidity burden of children, especially in developing countries, this scheme has been successful only in conjunction with other changes that have taken place in the transformation of rural communities' (Das et al. 2000).

A little while ago we discussed Calain's critique of the global surveillance system now being implemented. What kind of information should such systems aim to feed upwards? In much of the world there is little or no provision for the reporting of vaccine-related adverse events (Vaccine Safety Datalink Group 2005). Indeed, informal pressures or inadequate training may stand in the way of their being recorded by frontline health workers. But consider what a system for recording and reporting vaccine-related adverse events might offer. In much of the world there is no provision for parents who are convinced that their child has been adversely affected by a vaccine making the fact known. How is their concern then expressed? Sharing their conviction with friends and neighbours, or more widely and impersonally through the internet, may provide the basis for rumour, collective non-compliance, media attention, or legal action for damages. The lack of an institutionalised procedure for expressing anxieties or doubts, or for having them impartially investigated, can thus call other forms of expression into existence. The fate of the Indian HPV vaccine trials in Andhra Pradesh and Gujarat can serve both as a warning and as a guide to future practice.

The conclusion of much of the research summarised here is that immunisation programmes can only remain sustainable as donor funding is withdrawn if they stimulate active demand through building on local knowledge, capacities, and perceived needs. All of this suggests a metric of achievement very different from that which governs global health today. Why has this research seemingly had so little impact? What stands in the way? We return to this question in the final chapter of this book. Our discomforting sense, for the moment, is that the answer might lie far outside the field of public health.

A little more than a decade ago, James C. Scott, a leading authority on peasant societies, published a book with the subtitle *How Certain Schemes to Improve the Human Condition Have Failed* (Scott 1998). In the book, he compares a number of large-scale state projects in fields of urban planning and agriculture: projects in 'social engineering', he calls them. Part of Scott's purpose in writing the book, he explains, is to try to understand why large-scale essentially progressive and utopian schemes often failed those they were intended to benefit, and tragically so. The examples he uses do not come from the field of public health. Precisely for this reason, his conclusions give pause for reflection. 'What is perhaps most striking about high-modernist schemes . . . is how little confidence they repose in the skills, intelligence and experience of ordinary people'. He shows how highly functionalised planning can destroy people's inventiveness, local knowledge, and adaptability (Scott 1998, pp. 348–9). Scott argues for the importance of what he calls *metis*, knowledge that can only come from practical experience—the practical experience of living and working in a particular place at a particular time. Only institutions, schemes for human betterment that are infused by, and respect, this *metis* are likely to thrive and truly to improve people's lives.

Conclusions

Introduction of the rotavirus vaccine in African, Asian, and Latin American countries depended on supplies of the vaccine being transported safely from their sites of production, on recommendations from WHO being followed, and in many cases on funds being made available by the GAVI Alliance. The benefits of introduction of the vaccine for children's health, for the reduction of diarrhoea-related mortality and morbidity, depend on much more. National, and perhaps regional, health authorities have to ensure that vaccine supplies reach the communities in which at-risk children live. Health workers have to mobilise communities, ideally ensuring that rotavirus vaccination is combined with the other sanitary and dietary steps that communities need to take. Mothers in those communities have to be convinced, or coerced, into accepting vaccination for their child, although their understanding of the aetiology of diarrhoea may depart radically from that of biomedicine. At each step in this chain, from the global sites of production, expertise, and resource allocation to the local community, those responsible face conflicting pressures. Health policy-makers, for example, are under pressure to conform to international guidelines and rapidly to introduce new vaccines. But they may also have to face 'pressures from below', reflecting anxieties and concerns that, for whatever reason, have come to focus on vaccination. The tendency in global public health is to assume that advice from above will be followed, and where necessary to seek explanations of the 'deviant' behaviour of those who fail to comply. Our perspective in this book, rather differently, is to try to understand how, at each interface along the chain, those responsible seek to reconcile the pressures they face. The tendency in global health is also to measure success in terms of coverage or (increasingly) in terms of the number of countries having introduced a new vaccine. Here too our perspective is rather different. We suggest that the focus has to shift towards the creation of effective community demand: a far more challenging task. But only in this way can the long-term viability of vaccination programmes, and the long-term protection of children's health, be safeguarded. However, the pressures to conform to global priorities, and uncritically to follow standardised recommendations, are growing. We turn now to the global institutions in which policy is made and recommendations formulated. How do they exert pressure? On what basis does their authority rest?

Chapter 3

The global politics of health: actors and initiatives

Desmond McNeill, Steinar Andresen,
and Kristin Sandberg

Introduction

As previous chapters have shown, concern about the health of the world is hardly
new. What is new, especially in the last two decades, is the scale and influence of
major global initiatives such as the Global Fund to Fight HIV/AIDS, TB and
Malaria and—more specifically relating to immunisation—GAVI. These are, we
suggest, a mixed blessing. On the positive side, they bring increased attention and
substantial resources, leading to significant benefits for millions. Thanks to GAVI,
world leaders, powerful decision-makers, and indeed the public at large have
been made far more aware of the potential benefits that can be obtained by extending the coverage of existing vaccines and developing new ones, and massive financial resources have been devoted to this end, saving millions of children's lives.
Also, again thanks mainly to GAVI, a degree of unity and coordination has been
achieved between different actors at the global level. But there are negative aspects
also. The power that global actors have exerted, based primarily, although not
exclusively, on their financial resources, has exacerbated the asymmetric relations
that exist between strong and weak actors, threatening to reduce the already limited autonomy of the latter—most notably the governments of poorer countries.
There is a risk of homogeneous 'one size fits all' solutions being applied in all
countries, and also of national priorities—whether between health and other sectors, or within the health sector—being altered against the preferred choices of the
individual countries.

Although we are not questioning the intentions of global actors who contribute
to this situation, we do note that the effect of their actions is to strengthen the 'verticality' in the global health system. In this system—as noted in earlier chapters—
money, and vaccines themselves, emanate from the global level and travel down
from national to district to village levels, accompanied by technical advice,
exhortation, and targets to be achieved. In return—up the chain, emanating

from the most local level—come reports on performance and measures of achievements, expressed in terms of numbers of children vaccinated. In this way not only is the autonomy of national governments reduced, their accountability may even be reversed. Instead of being accountable 'downwards' to their citizens, they become accountable 'upwards' to global actors. In this chapter we shall show how this tendency has been exacerbated in recent years, as a result of an increased focus on numerical targets and 'results-based' assistance, closely associated with the huge influence of GAVI.

Associated with these processes, whether as cause or consequence (and the causal links are quite complex, as we will see), we find other tendencies in recent decades: a weakening of WHO, a greater role for the private sector, and increased emphasis on economics as the basis for priority-setting and for gaining political support for health initiatives.

The complex system with which we are concerned is composed of numerous actors, at global, national, and local levels, and with varying and sometimes conflicting interests. In this chapter we analyse the dynamics of this system, especially at the global level, although touching on the interaction between global and national levels. We start by examining the roles and influence of the main actors in the world of immunisation, asking: from where do they draw their power and authority? There have been significant changes during the last 20 years, especially owing to GAVI, and we devote much of the chapter to this important new alliance. We indicate the power of money as a 'vertical' force, strongly influencing national priorities and demanding accountability from nation states, but we also show how money, and more specifically the enormous start-up grant from the BMGF, significantly altered relations between key global actors.

In Chapter 1 we quoted the Report from the 1975 meeting of the UNICEF-WHO Joint Committee on Health Policy: 'It is of paramount importance that the major effort in the Programme must come from the individual countries concerned.' (JC20/UNICEF-WHO/75.4) But as years went by, the emphasis shifted more to providing finance, and this required attracting support for the sector. The adoption of UCI as the core of the Child Survival Revolution, which was favoured more by UNICEF than WHO, reflected the imperatives of attracting attention and resources. This was an important step in the move towards a more 'vertical' approach, bringing with it a greater need for measures and targets of performance. In a later section of this chapter we discuss at some length the problems that this gives rise to.

The ways in which WHO relates to countries may be divided into core functions and supportive functions (Jamison et al. 1998). Core functions address problems of the global commons, in this case the transborder risks of infectious disease. The failure of one country to control the spread of infectious diseases like polio or measles will have negative externalities for other countries, yet incentives to control spread are not sufficiently high for countries since they cannot fully reap the potential benefit. Hence the need for collective effort at the global level to *promote* international public goods (in this case immunisation), and to manage *surveillance* (of disease prevalence) and *control* (through increased immunisation coverage). These core functions, it is argued, serve all countries—rich and poor. Supportive functions, on the other hand, are activities that assist what is the primary responsibility of nation states. These functions are activated when the international community ' . . . mobilise resources such as knowledge and money to support countries with special development needs' (Jamison et al. 1998, p. 516). The intensity of such support varies according to need, and may span strategies from technical cooperation to capacity building and performance enhancement. Jamison et al. argue that supportive functions are inversely related to development: irrelevant for high-income countries, but essential for many low-income countries and countries in crisis.

Thus, whilst all countries are similar with respect to the core functions of WHO, affirming these through decisions within MoHs, they differ according to whether they require technical and financial assistance to meet the expectations of contributing to global immunisation goals. One may roughly divide countries into three groups with regard to immunisation: those that receive financial assistance, those that provide financial assistance, and those that are neither donors nor recipients, but self-sufficient in the way they handle their national immunisation programmes.

The WHO Constitution, adopted by the International Health Conference held in New York in 1946, established WHO as a specialised agency within the terms of Article 57 of the Charter of the United Nations. WHO was to have a number of functions, of which the four first are:

(*a*) to act as the directing and coordinating authority on international health work

(*b*) to establish and maintain effective collaboration with the United Nations, specialised agencies, governmental health administrations, professional groups, and such other organisations as may be deemed appropriate

(*c*) to assist governments, on request, in strengthening health services

(*d*) to furnish appropriate technical assistance and, in emergencies, necessary aid on the request or acceptance of governments.

The constitution was ratified by the first WHA, held in Geneva in 1948. Since then, according to some commentators, WHO has 'moved from being the unquestioned leader of international health to searching for its place in the contested world of global health' (Brown et al. 2006, p. 64). Certainly a number of other actors entered the global health scene, or enhanced their influence, in the decades following. These included international actors (such as GAVI), with which this chapter is primarily concerned, but also NGOs and pharmaceutical companies. Some commentators have gone so far as to claim that 'WHO's leadership role has passed to the far wealthier and more influential World Bank, and the WHO's mission has been dispersed among other UN agencies' (Silver 1998, p. 728, quoted in Brown et al. 2006). How can this situation have come about?

Sources of power and authority

In this section we analyse the sources of influence of the various actors on the global immunisation scene, using representation in the GAVI Board as criterion for inclusion in the list: governments of industrialised countries, international organisations, governments of developing countries, foundations, NGOs, research institutes, and vaccine manufacturers.

The power and authority of these actors derives from a range of different sources. In the global health arena the most important, perhaps more than ever today, is money. As shown by a recent review article in the Lancet (Ravishankar et al. 2009), the magnitude of development assistance to health has increased considerably in the last two decades. The number of actors, and sources of funds, has also increased considerably, leading to severe fragmentation (McCoy et al. 2009). Development assistance for health quadrupled from US$5·6 billion in 1990 to US$21·8 billion in 2007, doubling over the course of the first 11 years, and again in the next six. During this period, the relative contributions of different channels of assistance changed substantially (Ravishankar et al. 2009). The most substantial change was the percentage mobilised by the UN agencies (WHO, UNICEF, UNFPA, UNAIDS), which fell from 32·3% to 14·0%. The World Bank and regional banks peaked at 21·7% in 2000, falling back to 7·2% by 2007. The share from bilateral agencies decreased from 46·8% in 1990 to 34·0% in 2007. The massive increases in funding that account for this changed pattern came from other sources: the share of resources flowing through NGOs increased from 13·1% in 1990 to 24·9% in 2006. The Global Fund and GAVI scaled up from almost nothing to 8·3% and 4·2%, respectively, in 2007. And the proportion from the BMGF alone rose to 3·9% in 2007. The BMGF has increased global health commitments substantially since 2004, reaching nearly US$2 billion in both 2006 and 2007; a large share of their disbursements were transferred to the other channels of assistance listed above, including GAVI, the Global Fund, the World Bank, and UN agencies (Ravishankar et al. 2009). Of the total assistance, most was in the form of grants and loans, but a significant proportion (rising from about a third to almost half over the period) was in kind: drugs, medical supplies, and support to management, research, and technical assistance.

Another important source of authority is expertise, whose significance within the multilateral system has long been acknowledged (Haas 1990, 1992). There has been an upsurge of research on the topic in recent years (Bøås and McNeill 2004; Stone and Maxwell 2005), perhaps because the construction of expertise-based authority has been a conscious strategy of several multilateral organisations, particularly the World Bank, which since Wolfensohn's speech at their Annual Meeting in 1996 has attempted to purvey the image of being a 'knowledge bank'. In the global health arena one may distinguish between the expertise of health specialists and of economists. Decisions concerning priorities within the health sector, and more specifically with regard to immunisation, involve a complex mix of medical, economic, and political considerations. In recent decades there has been an increase in the authority of economic analysis as a basis for decision-making, in health as in many other fields. Internationally, this is perhaps most clearly manifested by the role of the World Bank, which, in 1987, published a report entitled *Financing Health Services in Developing Countries: An Agenda for Reform* (World Bank 1987). It followed this up with a World Development Report (the annual flagship report of the organisation) entitled *Investing in Health* (World Bank 1993). This made use of the concept which rapidly became very influential as a guide to decision-making: the disability-adjusted life year (DALY). This is a measure of overall disease burden, expressed as the number of years lost due to ill health, disability or early death. WHO followed suit, adopting the DALY approach in 2000. Under the leadership of Gro Harlem Brundtland, it also commissioned the Harvard economist Jeffrey Sachs to prepare the major study *Macroeconomics and Health: Investing in Health for Economic Development* (Sachs 2001). In international organisations, the logic of economics has become increasingly dominant and the expertise of economists has thereby become relatively more important. A similar process is apparent at national level in most countries, leading to greater power of the Ministry of Finance, relative to the MoH, and of economists within the latter.

A third source of authority is an actor's mandate: the extent to which it formally represents a group of actors (individuals, firms, countries etc.). In the global health arena, the obvious example is that of WHO. 'Of the global health actors only the WHO has the *formal-legal legitimacy* for the collective action of all states—it includes all nation states, small and large, weak and strong, rich and poor' (Kickbusch et al. 2010, p. 552).

In recent years there has been a burgeoning literature concerning the power and authority of international organisations (Cox 1997; Ruggie 1998; Barnett and Finnemore 2004), and as a result several other relevant factors could be added to this list, such as moral authority, leadership, convening power, access to wider networks, and the reputation that the actor has within developing countries. One source of power that is especially worth noting is related to what is known as 'performance legitimacy' (sometimes contrasted with 'process legitimacy'). Actors may gain legitimacy, irrespective of other sources, if they actually manage to achieve what are considered to be legitimate goals. This was a major driving force behind the promotion of public–private partnerships in the last decade. The point is elaborated on in Bull and McNeill (2007), which notes the power that the private sector derives from 'performance legitimacy'. The private sector is powerful not only directly as a market actor, but also as an idea. The belief that, subject as it is to market forces, the private sector is more efficient and effective than the public sector helps explain the appeal of 'public–private partnerships'. GAVI itself is one of the most striking examples of such public–private partnerships, and the crucial role that Bill Gates played was not merely in providing massive funding but also in emphasising the importance of performance, measured by concrete results. A former GAVI Executive Secretary stressed that 'GAVI is well positioned to take a leading role in providing lessons learned and new best practices in data quality and results-based financing programmes' (Lob-Levyt 2009, p. 209).

Against this background, we now briefly consider each actor in turn, assessing the sources of their power and authority, and how this may have changed in recent decades.

Governments of industrialised countries

The power of industrialised countries, in the context of global health and immunisation, derives primarily from the money they give. In the period 2002–2007, the USA was the largest donor of development assistance to health, followed by the UK, Japan, Germany, France, the Netherlands, Canada, Sweden, Norway, and Italy (Ravishankar et al. 2009). These funds may be provided directly, as bilateral aid, currently accounting for about one-third of total development assistance to health, as noted above, but also indirectly when they finance international organisations. In the GAVI Alliance, the money from both is pooled. Industrialised countries may also derive some limited power and authority from their expertise, whether as health specialists or economists. This expertise may be manifested, for example, through their participation in international meetings or in documents produced by them.

As discussed below, within GAVI there have been notable changes over time: in the early years donor countries gave massive support while exercising only limited influence, but they have subsequently become much more active and influential in the setting of policy. The USA and some European countries have been the most influential of these actors. There have been differences in emphasis between the two, notably over the issue of support to health systems, with Norway especially emphasising their importance in an effective national immunisation system. These to some extent follow earlier tensions between Europe and America over the CVI, which some, especially the Dutch and Nordic countries, felt was too American a project, and too focused on finding technological solutions for health problems in developing countries (Muraskin 2005).

International organisations

WHO, UNICEF, and the World Bank are the major three international organisations of relevance. The power and authority of WHO derive primarily from the formal–legal legitimacy granted by its mandate, noted above, and its expertise. But as economic expertise has gradually grown in influence by comparison with public health, the latter has perhaps become of lesser significance. Kickbusch et al. (2010) note that WHO has been able to benefit not only from these but also its moral standing, which 'has always been an absolutely essential source of legitimacy for the WHO' (Kickbusch et al. 2010, p. 553). However, according to the same source: 'in the 1990s WHO was pushed into the frame of a development organization and began to compete for funding of programs with the many other actors; as a result, for a period it lost much of its influence and strategic purpose' (Kickbusch et al. 2010, p. 556).

In financial terms WHO is weak, with a budget of less than US$4 billion (2012–2013) of which the core budget from assessed contributions (i.e. untied funding) is only about US$1 billion dollars. By contrast, the BMGF annual budget for global health is about US$2 billion dollars. Over time, the power of WHO has gradually declined. But in the immunisation field, the situation following GAVI was complex: WHO became less influential relative to others, but benefited from playing a central role in this very important initiative. More recently it has perhaps lost out as GAVI became almost an organisation in itself, with WHO as something of a subcontractor.

UNICEF's mandate is clearly important as a source of formal authority— albeit overlapping somewhat with that of WHO. And UNICEF, arguably even more than WHO, derives moral authority from the close association between immunisation and the well-being of children. UNICEF was the spearhead of the universal immunisation campaign during the 1980s, in tandem with WHO.

As the goal of 80% coverage of the world's children was declared in 1990, the organisation changed its policy to one where countries should increasingly take responsibility for their own immunisation programmes, maintaining the delivery systems that UNICEF had invested in a decade earlier, and by 1998 UNICEF funding for immunisation was only a quarter of what it had been in 1990 (Gauri and Khaleghian 2002). UNICEF also derives authority from its expertise in vaccine procurement and delivery. It has long been the principal vaccine procurement agency for many countries, has provided equipment for cold chains, and has supported social mobilisation for immunisation. Financially, UNICEF is better placed than WHO, but less well-endowed than the World Bank. Changes over time have been due mainly to the varying extent to which UNICEF itself has prioritised vaccination: from a high level (with UCI), then moving away from immunisation as a priority, and more recently perhaps moving back again.

The World Bank derives power and authority primarily from the money that it has at its disposal and the expertise of its staff—most notably in economics. The World Bank has been increasing its influence over global and regional health policies since the 1980s (Calain 2006a, p. 6; citing also Walt 2001). By the early 1990s the World Bank was the world's leading external financier of health in low-income countries and 'became prominent in developing international health policy and strategy', but 'since 2000, the Bank's dominance in health has arguably shrunk. Its lending to the health sector has fallen by one-third' (People's Health Movement 2008, p. 280). Before GAVI, the World Bank had only a limited involvement in the immunisation field. Thanks to its membership of the Alliance this changed; but now its efforts are largely focused on health systems.

Other international organisations have played a much less significant role. UNDP, which along with the World Bank is often credited with convening power, was a member of the CVI Standing Committee, but it has not been a major actor in the immunisation field.

Governments of developing countries

The primary power and authority of developing countries in the context of immunisation programmes derives from the sovereignty they exercise over their people and their territory, which external actors are obliged to recognise. In practice, the extent of this power varies considerably; here, as in other fields of development assistance, countries that are financially very dependent on aid have much less power. To what extent can a developing country resist the intrusion of an outside actor, should it wish to do so? It is relevant to distinguish here between a country's decisions regarding the allocation of financial and human resources, and regarding more technical health-related issues such as the introduction of a new vaccine. With regard to the former, it is from its financial resources that a country derives its power; if these are limited, as in say Malawi or Nepal, the power of the 'donor' is much greater. It is worth noting that according to WHO estimates 23 countries have over 30% of their total health expenditures funded by donors, and although aid accounts for only 0.3% of total expenditures on health globally, the figure is 6.5% in subSaharan Africa (Sridhar 2010, p. 459).

With regard to more technical issues, external actors can be relatively powerful. WHO, by virtue both of its mandate and its expertise, enjoys a high degree of authority in the health field. The extent to which a country can question WHO recommendations or advice depends on the level of medical expertise in the country concerned. While Malawi and Nepal, for example, are here at a disadvantage, countries such as India and Brazil, by contrast, are strong. If they wish they can to a far greater extent than weak states exert their power to challenge and if necessary resist outside actors (see Chapter 4). Over the past two decades or so the power and authority of developing countries has not changed much. However, as discussed below, there is evidence that 'weak' countries may now have even less autonomy as a result of GAVI.

Foundations

Private foundations have always played an important role in international health, with the Rockefeller Foundation as perhaps the most influential and active for much of the 20th century. Rockefeller played an important role in the CVI and later became a member of the GAVI Board. Although they may accumulate moral authority, as the Rockefeller Foundation certainly did, foundations derive their power mainly from their money and perhaps expertise (Bull and McNeill 2007). The extraordinarily large grant to GAVI by the BMGF makes this a rather unusual case; money has here clearly been very important. But so too has moral authority; saving children's lives is akin to a crusade, and a person or charitable foundation that takes up this cause may thereby exercise considerable moral authority, which can be used to persuade others to devote resources to this purpose. The BMGF funds not only GAVI, but also other organisations (WB, WHO, UNICEF, even USAID) as well as vaccine research and development, trials, and supply.

Non-governmental organizations

Although they have both money and expertise, a relatively more important source of power of NGOs is moral authority. In some contexts they derive power from their claim to represent a constituency, especially if they are organisations with large numbers of members, but this is less relevant in the present context. They may also derive power from their participation in networks, both formal and informal. One specialised NGO, the Programme for Appropriate Technology in Health (PATH), played a very important role leading up to, and during, the establishment of GAVI—thanks, one might argue, largely to expertise and personal contacts. PATH was founded in 1977 as the Program for the Introduction and Adaptation of Contraceptive Technology (PIACT), but has been known as PATH since 1981. It is based in Seattle, the home of the BMGF, and according to its vice-president Michael Free: 'I think we could say that PATH originated the concept of public–private partnerships, long before it became cachet' (Programme for Appropriate Technology in Health 2012). It is still a significant actor, receiving four out of the 20 largest individual grants from the BMGF in the period 1999–2007, totaling US$353 million (People's Health Movement 2008, p. 246). Chris Elias, head of PATH, announced in 2011 that he was leaving, after a decade, to take over as head of the global development program at the BMGF. Other NGOs have been less important, but do play a role, for example Save the Children.

Research organisations

The source of power of medical research organisations in this specialised field obviously derives from their expertise. In view of the fervour with which some of them promote the cause one could argue that they also have moral authority. Among universities, Johns Hopkins University Bloomberg School of Public Health and the London School of Hygiene and Tropical Medicine have been particularly prominent. The combination of scientific expertise and concern for social justice that characterises many members of this group gives them considerable influence in the 'epistemic community' that promotes new vaccines (see section 'Changing relations between global actors: the impact of GAVI').

Vaccine producers

The firms that produce vaccines derive their power from being suppliers of a specialised product, requiring considerable expertise, and as holders of patents based on many years of research and testing. The market has until recently been dominated by a few very large international companies, but now, in part thanks to GAVI, the situation is changing. A few vaccine producers, in countries such as India, Brazil, and Indonesia, are starting to compete with 'big pharma' in regional and, increasingly, global markets. Although information about production costs is carefully guarded, making it difficult for the purchasers of vaccines to drive a hard bargain, the growing number of producers has clearly increased the degree of competition in what is a rather unusual market. Critics argue, however, that the failure of GAVI to deliver the substantial price reductions that were promised is evidence of the continued market power of these firms. What is new, under GAVI, is the closer collaboration between vaccine producers and other actors, especially WHO. Their participation in the GAVI Board is the most obvious manifestation of this. It is not clear that this gives them significantly more power than before, but one might argue that it gives them increased legitimacy—and perhaps more influence over global decision-making in this field.

Changing relations between global actors: the impact of GAVI

In this section we focus primarily on relations between the three main international organisations—WHO, UNICEF, and the World Bank—and the impact of GAVI. Among international development organisations, broadly defined, there is a complex collaborative/competitive relationship. They share a common goal—whether the increased welfare of the poor or a more specific aim such as reduced child mortality—but they are usually competing for funds, and influence, with other agencies (Bøås and McNeill 2004; McNeill and Lera St Clair 2009). Against this background, the impact of GAVI is interesting because of what it achieved (much better collaboration between WHO, UNICEF, and the World Bank) and how it achieved it (mainly by virtue of its strength in financial terms). This collaboration between major actors contrasted starkly with the period immediately before, which ended with the demise of the CVI. The result has been that GAVI itself has become a major actor, and its approach to immunisation has become very influential.

In analysing the situation, in broad terms, there are two particularly important and related relationships to consider. One is between WHO and other international organisations—notably UNICEF and the World Bank. The other is between these organisations and the private sector. The two issues are related because while some international organisations, most notably the World Bank, are very willing to work with the private sector, WHO has been reluctant to do so. This, combined with 'turf battles', led to poor relations between these bodies: a situation which paved the way for GAVI.

When GAVI was created in 1999, it signalled a new era in global health cooperation: an innovative funding and collaborative mechanism, and a striking example of what was happening across the board, in particular regarding infectious diseases. The multilateral organisations and donor countries embraced the idea of public–private partnerships as a means of meeting the new challenges of cooperation and leveraging more funds. The initial and crucial funding commitment of US$750 million from the BMGF was, during Phase 1, more than matched by rich country governments, such that donor contributions by the end of this period totaled US$1.67 billion (Chee et al. 2008).

GAVI emerged against a backdrop of resource scarcity and doubts about the capacity of WHO and UNICEF to deliver on child immunisation. In brief, the two organisations, especially WHO, were increasingly lacking in 'performance legitimacy' and as a result losing in the battle for funding. As elaborated on elsewhere, doubts were voiced towards the end of the 1990s by a broad range of individuals working with immunisation whether as scientists, advocates, or policy-makers (Bull and McNeill 2007; Sandberg et al. 2010). Blame was directed largely at WHO, and forces were gathering around proposals for a renewed effort. The CVI, which had been launched after the World Summit for Children in September 1990, was widely regarded as unsuccessful and underfunded. It had tried, largely without success, to bridge the gap between public and private sectors (Muraskin 2002, p. 116). The CVI 'fought for years to maintain its relative independence from the World Health Organization' but 'was de facto absorbed into WHO' (Muraskin 2002, p. 124). Distrust in the CVI was related to the two interconnected issues identified above. Regarding relations between the public and private sector, Muraskin (2005, pp. 27–28) notes that:

> Bringing members of the public and private sectors together constituted a daunting challenge for the CVI. There existed a great gulf of distrust, often bordering on outright contempt, among people in the two sectors. . . . The idea that the profit motive should play a key role in determining which lifesaving vaccines were produced was seen as fundamentally immoral; vaccines should be a public service, even a public right, not something bought and sold.

Relations were scarred following the controversial issue of private sector involvement in the development of a heat-resistant polio vaccine (Muraskin 2002, pp. 121–123), and WHO's scepticism of the private sector was reciprocated: 'many industry leaders had strongly negative feelings towards WHO' (Muraskin 2002, p. 136). Relations with other international organisations were also not easy. The WHO had a reputation of tending always to be the dominant party in cooperative arrangements—unwilling to have equal partners in international health efforts. Senior WHO officials at the time of GAVI establishment adhered to a strong organisational culture—that WHO was the lead UN agency in health and should not follow the initiatives of other actors. WHO was sceptical of the World Bank and feared that they would take an active role in immunisation. This possibility was welcomed by some others; indeed, at the end of the 1990s 'It was assumed by many observers that the Bank was making a bid for leadership in the vaccine area because the WHO had continued to fail in that area' (Muraskin 2002, p. 142). But authoritative sources, cited by Muraskin, make it clear that this was not in fact a real alternative. The World Bank 'had neither the desire nor ability to take leadership in health or immunization away from the WHO' (Muraskin 2002, p. 143). Both the World Bank and industry representatives were, however, dissatisfied with existing vaccination programmes and the fact that the introduction of new vaccines had lost momentum.

Dr Gro Harlem Brundtland took up office as WHO Director-General in 1998. She appointed a small group of senior policy advisers, headed by Jonas Gahr Store, also from Norway. They arrived at a critical time. The termination of CVI was announced by WHO at a meeting in Bellagio, Italy (Chee et al. 2008, p. 25), which in fact marked the transition from CVI to GAVI, but the path was initially not smooth. As the idea of GAVI was developing in 1998, representatives from WHO, UNICEF, the World Bank, the Rockefeller Foundation, and the International Federation of Pharmaceutical Manufacturers & Associations (IFPMA) formed a Working Group. Participants in the group at the time state that the internal dynamic of the group was shaped by the fact that most members knew each other well; several had been active participants in the CVI. Over time, several had moved out of WHO, but continued to work on the same issues in other organisations.

The majority of the Working Group members wanted GAVI to focus primarily on new vaccine introduction. WHO and UNICEF representatives, however, argued that the final recommendations of the group did not reflect opinions expressed at the wider consultations with donor and recipient countries. This difference prevailed for a year, as described by a senior professional who knew both CVI and WHO well:

> In some ways, there is a tension in the international health area, the vaccine area, that is never going to be resolved. And it is the tension between using new science quickly, where you can use it, and the desire on the part of immunization practitioners, the people more involved at the country level, to get the basic vaccines to everybody.

A second and more political tension between the stakeholders was the organisational structure of the emerging initiative: should it be an independent organisation or an alliance? WHO broke off negotiations as pressures intensified towards GAVI becoming an independent organisation because, according to senior WHO officials at the time, 'we felt that these actors (the World Bank, industry and American stakeholders) were taking a public health mandate out of WHO'. 'In the end', however, a CVI observer noted, 'GAVI became a compromise between the impatience in the World Bank, industry and some of these actors, and the demands of UNICEF and WHO that a new initiative had to fit a framework that the UN organizations could accept'.

In the negotiation phase leading to GAVI, the WHO leadership explain that they insisted that GAVI should be an alliance and not an independent organisation. A crucial element in breaking the deadlock that followed was the prospect of large increases in funding on the horizon. According to a representative of the WHO leadership team: 'when Gates came up with enormous sums, we could choose to be principled or pragmatic. We chose the latter. Our attitude was to do the utmost to engage them.' According to several key actors, there were signs as early as 1998 that the BMGF might be willing to fund a new global initiative on immunisation.

A variety of sources, including our own interviews, agree that in the early years of GAVI an unusually high degree of trust was established between the members of the Working Group. For example

> GAVI constituted a remarkable innovation in institutional terms, in that it managed to a considerable extent to overcome the limitations of the international organizations concerned (turf battles, and slow-moving bureaucracy), achieving instead good collaboration and rapid and effective action. An important contributing factor to this achievement was a small group of very able and highly committed individuals, willing to set aside narrow institutional interests and act in a spirit of 'constructive ambiguity. (Chee et al. 2008)

As noted above, members of the group were selected mainly on the basis of their knowledge of immunisation, and several of them knew each other well from having worked together in the CVI. A few key individuals played an important role in the effective operation of the Working Group, most notably Tore Godal, who was appointed by the heads of the founding partners as leader of the Working Group and Executive Secretary of the emerging alliance in June 1999 (Sandberg et al. 2010). They could be described as members of an 'epistemic community', as defined by Haas (1992, p. 3): 'An epistemic community is a network of professionals with recognized expertise and competence in a particular domain and an authoritative claim to policy-relevant knowledge within that domain or issue-area.' Although all four of Haas' criteria for identifying an epistemic community are relevant, it is perhaps the first that is most striking in this case: 'a shared set of normative and principled beliefs, which provide a value-based rationale for the social action of community members' (Haas 1992). Certainly the Working Group shared a common purpose, in some cases passionately so. But there is no doubt that money played a crucial role in bringing about the necessary organisational change. An evaluation report includes a quote from an anonymous commentator that expresses quite starkly the background to GAVI and the crucial role of the new funding:

> ... the $100 million commitment for CVP at Path from the Gates Foundation followed by the establishment of the Global Fund for Children's Vaccine ($750 million over 5 years) was the tipping point that made everything else possible. (Chee et al. 2008, p. 249)

Established in 1998 as a forum to agree aims and objectives for the alliance, the Working Group was characterised by some as the 'heart of GAVI'. It was made up of technical personnel from the partner organisations and, until it ended in 2008, it played a crucial role in negotiating collaboration (Muraskin 2005, p. 104). On the Governing Board were high-level leaders of the partner organisations, with the Chair position rotating between the heads of WHO and UNICEF. There was also a small secretariat which, during the first 5 years, worked in the basement of the Geneva UNICEF office. With hindsight, one might suggest that this modest size was an advantage: the coordinating hub was so small that this newcomer could not possibly take over the role of the GAVI partner agencies.

Compromises needed to be reached on a number of issues, and it is instructive to identify a few of these to see how they map onto the different actors involved: both the lead organisations—WHO, UNICEF, and the World Bank—and some other actors. We may briefly consider three:

- Attitudes to the vaccine industry: should they be kept at arm's length?
- Should development of new vaccines be prioritised over the wider distribution of existing vaccines?
- Should investment in vaccines be prioritised over improving health systems?

Attitudes to the vaccine industry: WHO, historically, certainly adhered to the view that they should they be kept at arm's length. The World Bank disagreed. Of the other actors, the vaccine industry itself was of course the most important; they wanted to be involved but, as noted above, did not trust WHO.

Should development of new vaccines be prioritised over the distribution of existing vaccines even more widely? Here the dividing lines did not run simply between organisations; within WHO itself there were the 'bench guys' and the 'bush guys', in their own parlance (Bull and McNeill 2007, p. 72) In UNICEF, the latter group (those who spent time in the field) was more strongly represented. Among other actors, opinions varied, but potential conflict was considerably muted by the fact that the massive funding offered by GAVI allowed the possibility that there would be more money for both new and existing vaccines.

Should investment in vaccines be prioritised over improving health systems? This had long been, and remained, a source of disagreement, also between donor countries, with vaccine researchers and industry largely favouring the former. (Even within WHO and UNICEF there were differing views: 'bush guys' tending to favour the latter.) This issue is taken up again later in this chapter.

Partly owing to differing views about these issues, attitudes to GAVI within WHO and UNICEF were not uniformly positive. Members of the WHO leadership in the start-up phase of GAVI say in interviews that they experienced substantial resistance to the idea of a broader partnership on key immunisation objectives. They therefore saw their task as convincing the technical divisions of the benefits and potential of GAVI, and they adopted a pragmatic argument, clearly recognising the power of the purse. As one senior official put it in an interview: 'When would the WHO's influence be greater: if it owned two thirds of a large enterprise, or owning all of an enterprise that was half the size?'

At UNICEF, too, the leadership's support for GAVI contrasted with reluctance from the parts of the organisation directly involved with immunisation. In interviews in 2008, with the benefit of hindsight, observers note UNICEF's role as one of the paradoxes in the GAVI structure that 'the organization which was most involved with the delivery of vaccines to begin with, was opposed to the new situation that GAVI brought about.'

Within quite a short period of time GAVI grew. As it became more well-established it changed—some believe for the worse. A GAVI-commissioned study in 2002 described the Working Group as a 'crucially important element of the GAVI architecture . . . (having borne an) . . . exceptionally, perhaps unacceptably heavy burden of work', but asserted the need for GAVI to move ' . . . from a voluntary group of officials to a more business-like, managed system' (Caines and N'jie 2002, p. ii). GAVI grew considerably in terms of staff numbers, and changed its governance structure, its character, its leader, and to some extent its role. Features of this shift included:

– increases in the size and roles and responsibilities of the Secretariat . . .

– the development of more formal governance arrangements. (CEPA, 2010: 8)

Some of the individuals most closely concerned express regrets about the change, for two main reasons well summarised by a former WHO Working Group member, interviewed in 2008: 'The Working Group was really the heart of the alliance. With it, the alliance dies. GAVI is now an organization . . . and taking over many of the WHO functions in countries, in terms of interaction with countries and technical advice'. According to the same interviewee, almost a quarter of WHO's vaccine budget is GAVI funded, and donor countries have chosen largely to channel their support through GAVI. A second former Working Group member confirms this view in 2008: 'Now, GAVI is an entity. The governance structure changed. . . . They wanted to dampen and control the working group, and a more advisory role for the task forces. Much more power to the secretariat. More professional reporting, more professional management. Partners are now sub-contracting.' Several interviewees asserted that WHO had come to feel like a GAVI subcontractor, with implications for the organisation's priorities. For example:

> My biggest fear is our dependence on GAVI. It is skewed in a direction to areas that we would normally not pay so much attention to. New vaccines is getting the weight of the funding. The attention to the routine programme is being lost.

An interviewee from PATH asserted in 2008 that WHO felt threatened, but 'On the other hand, though, WHO has total authority in countries.' This is confirmed by a former Working Group member, but with reservations: 'WHO and UNICEF continue technical support at country level, but it is GAVI that funds it to do so. . . . The WHO position is weakened by being directly funded by GAVI'. In brief, GAVI itself has become like an organisation, with very considerable power, while relations between WHO, UNICEF, and the World Bank may be returning to 'normal'.

Against this backdrop, GAVI embarked on the first phase (2000–2005) of its mission: 'saving children's lives and protecting people's health through the widespread use of safe vaccines', funding basic children's immunisation in 70 low-income countries, introducing new combination vaccines that also included protection against new diseases, and supporting countries' immunisation services through a performance-based reward system (Chee et al. 2008). According to WHO estimates, this has been a remarkably successful endeavour: for the period 2000–2008, GAVI support is said to have prevented a cumulative 3.4 million future deaths, protected a cumulative 50.9 million children with basic vaccines against DTP3 (diphtheria, tetanus, and pertussis), and protected a cumulative 213 million children with new and underused vaccines.

The remarkable achievement of the GAVI initiative was to break up a logjam in the multilateral system; to change relations between key actors, such that they were able to work effectively together towards a common goal. It may be, as some critics claim, that the achievements of GAVI—the number of children vaccinated, the number of lives saved—have been exaggerated (Lim et al. 2008) or that more of its resources should have been put into building up health systems. Nevertheless, there can be no doubt that GAVI has huge achievements to its credit. One important respect in which GAVI has, at least so far, been generally unsuccessful is in reducing vaccine prices, although expectations here may have been 'misguided' (Chee et al. 2008, p. 84). But GAVI was surely a considerable achievement in institutional terms. Even if GAVI has now become more bureaucratic, less light on its feet, it did for a period manage to break out of the straightjacket that usually constrains efforts in the multilateral arena and for this it deserves full credit, as do the few highly committed professionals who played such a crucial part in its early years.

Thanks to its success in this regard, GAVI established 'performance legitimacy', thus gaining the confidence of donor countries, which were therefore willing to commit massive funding. (The alliance is highly praised by, for example, the International Task Force on Public Goods (Lele et al. 2005).) Rich countries were faced with a dilemma: wanting to disburse large amounts of funds to a good global cause, but not trusting the main multilateral organisations mandated to carry out the job, and which they themselves had established and, to a large extent, still controlled. GAVI offered them a solution, at least in the short run. The result was the increased influence of GAVI by comparison with, most notably, WHO.

In summary, GAVI has had a huge impact on global immunisation. The sheer volume of its resources not only enabled the scale of activities to increase enormously, it also had two other effects—which may or may not be lasting. One, described in some detail in the foregoing, was to improve the 'horizontal' relations between the main actors involved at global level. A second effect, we suggest, was to increase the 'verticality' in the system. This has long been a controversial issue. Feachem and Sabot (2006, p. 539), discussing the approach of the Global Fund, refer to it as 'the latest manifestation of the so-called vertical versus horizontal debate, which has consumed the global-health community for years' (see also Oliveira-Cruz et al. 2003). Kickbusch et al. (2010, p. 556) note that while many new health initiatives and actors have put health high on the global development agenda, many analyses have recently shown that they have 'reinforced the verticalization of approaches to resolve global health challenges'. This 'vertical' approach promotes a system in which the flow of funds from top down needs to be complemented by a flow of information from the bottom up: statistics of performance required by the donors in order to monitor and evaluate achievements, so as to provide the necessary evidence to secure continued funding. In the next section we consider vertical relations, and more specifically those between global actors and the nation states that receive donor funds.

Relations between the global and the national levels

Despite a rhetoric of 'country ownership', donor agencies have always tended to exercise considerable influence over health, and other policies, in countries receiving development assistance. This has been especially the case in countries most heavily dependent on aid. Thus a poor African country, for example, although being a member of WHO or UNICEF, and a shareholder in the World Bank, is also to some extent 'dominated' by them: dependent on their expert knowledge and financial resources. To quote a former Minister of Health in Mozambique: 'At the international level, a constant deluge of new initiatives, focusing on specific diseases or issues makes it extremely difficult for governments to develop and implement sound national health plans for their countries. . . . That is a crisis right now—the international community is not accepting developing country leadership.' (Global Economic Governance 2008, p. 1). GAVI has been criticised for contributing to this situation. Milstein et al. (2008, p. 5300) refer to priorities being 'perceived as highly globally driven by GAVI and the FTF [Financial Task Forces] resulting in limited regional and country ownership to the process'. Thus GAVI itself has, in recent years, become increasingly like an international organisation. Thanks to the power of the purse, GAVI can exercise power and authority over developing countries, and even, to some extent, over WHO and UNICEF.

Relations of power and authority become particularly apparent at the interface between the different actors when they meet—either literally in person or more indirectly though written communications. As part of our study, we occasionally had the opportunity to attend, as observers, meetings between key global actors. Such opportunities provided valuable insights into the relationships between them. One such event was a meeting entitled the *New and Under-utilized Vaccines Introduction (NUVI) Retreat*, which the lead author of this chapter was permitted to attend as an observer. It took place at UNICEF New York on 16 February 2009. The following description of the one-day event serves both to illustrate the nature of relations between key actors and to offer a small piece of empirical evidence supporting our argument.

The meeting in New York was for staff from UNICEF and WHO together with selected partners, and its purpose was to share and compare experience across regions and identify major issues. As the name 'retreat' implies, it was less formal than an official meeting, with time for relaxed discussion between attendees, many of whom knew each other quite well. (Since 2009 these retreats have taken place at 6-monthly intervals. They are normally held in, or near, either Geneva or New York—the headquarters of WHO and UNICEF, respectively—thus maintaining an equal balance between WHO and UNICEF).

The morning session in February 2009 was chaired by UNICEF with WHO as rapporteur. Expressing the equal standing of the two organisations, the roles were reversed in the afternoon. At the end of the day a closed meeting, to which observers were not invited, took place.

The majority of participants were from UNICEF and WHO: about 10 from each, with roughly equal numbers from headquarters and the regions. Others attending were the US CDC (four representatives), PATH (three), Johns Hopkins University Bloomberg School of Public Health (one), the Hib Initiative (one), Immunization BASICS (one), GAVI (two), and the BMGF (one). The discussion at the meeting was formally 'framed' in two respects: first, by the agenda itself, and second by the fact that those who reported were given a specified template to follow. The agenda may be seen as falling into three activities: learning, reporting, and planning/committing:

Learning: In principle, and generally in practice, this activity manifested an equal relationship between those who had similar experience (although of course their degree of experience and extent of expertise might vary).

Reporting: This appeared as a more hierarchical relationship, with those from the regional offices reporting not just to each other but to others who perhaps had some authority over them.

Planning/committing: This activity appeared as in part a hierarchical relationship; while it in a sense implies simply the provision of information, it also implies a commitment to deliver and to report at some future date on whether one has fulfilled this commitment.

In summary, the meeting primarily took the form of exchange of experiences, ideas, and plans; but there was also certainly an element of reporting on performance, implicitly hierarchical in nature.

As noted, those presenting their reports were required to do so according to a specified 'template':

- Status of introduction of new vaccines: HiB, pneumococcal vaccine, and rotavirus
- Technical assistance
- Surveillance of new and underutilised vaccines
- Impediments and solutions
- Priorities for next 6–12 months.

At the end of the meeting, the representative of the BMGF, who until then had not taken a very active part, gave some comments, expressing satisfaction with the proceedings in a way which suggested that this was, in practice, a very authoritative figure, and that an important purpose of the event, even if not explicitly stated, was to satisfy the BMGF.

A few excerpts from the discussion are particularly revealing. Several of those presenting took up the issue of what they called 'political will'. In practice, this seemed to be a code word for the unwelcome fact that some governments, such as India, are reluctant to approve and advocate the vaccines concerned. This raised the issue of how to achieve 'country ownership' of policies, i.e. to have countries agree to adopting new vaccines. One participant asked what to do when a country says 'We are not going to accept': 'Do we accept that? Is there a point at which we do . . . or do we never give up?' The comment from the Chair—'You don't need to answer that'—was met with laughter from the participants: a clear indication that this was a touchy subject.

Another point at which there was laughter was when the issue of payment for vaccines arose: 'How do we handle countries that cannot co-finance?' It was clear that this was a major problem in Africa, and a source of embarrassment, but no solution was forthcoming.

In general, the discussions were very amicable. One of the few issues which led to signs of tension or irritation concerned the use of evidence, especially modelling. One representative from a regional WHO office said: 'Modeling has a role. But we are using modeling to show people there is a problem (which they don't see). Then we use modeling again to show we are right. How to do it in a way that appears real to the country?' Another responded that 'Models do not create diseases that are not there.' Another argued that as long as the model is based on some empirical data—maybe from a different country—it is okay. The first speaker asserted that countries need 'something they can relate to. So it doesn't look like some numbers you are throwing at them.'

Following this there was also discussion about how to present data. One person commented that 'One of the most unseemly public health practices is parceling out deaths by disease'. Referring to a *Lancet* pie chart on the mortality of under-5s, someone said 'It looks as if vaccine-preventable diseases are no longer a problem.' What is needed is 'a pie-graph that shows much better how mortality can be prevented by vaccines'; from looking at this pie-graph 'immunisation seems to be a problem of the past'. The response was: 'Just make a new pie chart. We can make it visible.'

A member from WHO headquarters stressed the importance of cost-effectiveness models. 'You need to convince decision-makers. The models are too complicated, and build in assumptions which are not ours. . . . We are not controlling the models anymore.' (The implication was that industry does control such models.)

It is relevant to reflect on the message and its communication. The message—obviously, given the purpose of the meeting—is that countries must commit to adopting new vaccines and to increasing coverage of underused vaccines. More interesting is the issue of how to get the message across. It was clear from the meeting that advocacy and carefully crafted evidence were important, but that these are controversial. It was also clear that while the message was being conveyed 'down' the system, demands were being made for reports on progress and performance 'up' the system.

As noted, the meeting was amicable and constructive—an example of good collaboration between like-minded professionals with a shared purpose. Decisions or conclusions were not forced on unwilling parties. But the issues discussed, and especially those which gave rise to some discomfort, were somewhat revealing of the very varying power and authority, not only of those attending the meeting but also, perhaps even more so, of those not attending the meeting—representatives of governments, some of which are hugely dependent on global funding and are required to satisfy the demands of those who provide financial and other forms of assistance.

Evidence, decision-making, and reporting

All countries that receive assistance are to some extent subject to pressure and control from those that provide it, the extent being rather closely correlated with the degree of dependence on such funding (which may be crudely measured by the proportion of their health budget that is externally funded). This power is especially manifest with regard to establishing priorities (for example how much emphasis is to be placed on immunisation) and to the reporting on performance that is required (what is reported, how, and to whom). This promotes an economic–technocratic perspective, and tends to give power and authority to those individuals and organisations that adopt such a perspective. Quantification plays a very significant part in such an approach, whether in estimating disease incidence and the costs of ill health (used in social cost-benefit analysis for setting priorities) or assessing performance based on, for example, numbers of children vaccinated.

Thus, as the encounter described in the previous section suggests, numbers are important in two respects. First, in relation to decision-making: on what basis should the priority to be given to vaccines, as opposed to other uses of scarce healthcare resources, be made? Second, in relation to reporting: why, how, and to whom are reports on performance due?

Should vaccines be the highest priority for expenditure within the health sector or, where resources are very limited, should they be better spent on, say, curative medicine, or on improving the health system, or on other preventive measures such as improved water supply and sanitation? (The debate is complicated by the fact that these are in part complementary, i.e. that effective vaccine delivery is dependent on good health systems.) A wider issue is the priority of health expenditure in relation to other sectors, but it may be assumed that the relevant audience here is one which is primarily concerned with promoting health. (To complicate matters, there has been some discussion in the literature as to whether aid to the health sector leads to a diversion of a government's own funds to other sectors, but the evidence is not conclusive (Batniji and Bendavid 2012).)

It is apparent that governments receiving development assistance funds for the health sector, especially from GAVI, have been influenced not only by the promise of massive funding but also by the imperative of applying arguments based on the use of a rather clearly specified economic analysis, requiring detailed quantitative estimates of impacts, costs, and benefits. This focus on quantifiable costs and benefits is linked to the increasing dominance of economic analysis in international organisations, including WHO, that was noted above. Commenting on the WHO-commissioned report *Macroeconomics and Health: Investing in Health for Economic Development*, Waitzkin (2003) argues that the authors shifted the prevailing emphasis from the social determinants of health, such as inequality in income, class, and power, to investment in health in support of economic growth, and that the focus on economic productivity in the report 'diminishes the importance of health as a fundamental human right'. In his view health was no longer invested in as an entitlement (Waitzkin 2003, p. 361). Labonté and Gagnon (2010) is even more critical, arguing that this economic approach is driven by donor self-interest that may or may not reflect local health needs. This, they argue, explains why non-communicable diseases rank low in the aid and development discourse: chronic disease is less of a threat to national or global transborder health security than infectious disease.

Even if one sets aside the concerns of Waitzkin and Labonté and Gangon, the economic approach to priority setting has other limitations. Apart from uncertainties as to how costs and benefits are to be valued, there are sources of uncertainty that lie outside the realm of economics. One of these is the question of vaccine safety. This is a technical issue, requiring the expertise of virologists, immunologists, and epidemiologists. It is very often also a controversial political issue. A government may be convinced of the merits of a vaccine, but encounter strong popular resistance that perhaps cannot (and, we would add, should not) be ignored. Examples of precisely this are to be found throughout this book.

How does resistance, at national level, to the introduction of a new vaccine manifest itself? Perhaps the most obvious is simply to refuse offers of assistance. But, as indicated above, donors can be rather insistent. GAVI not only offers assistance in the form of vaccines, and advice concerning vaccines, but also assistance in preparing requests for vaccines. Thus a consultant might be paid by GAVI to prepare a request to GAVI on behalf of a national government. The latter might indeed be keen to have GAVI support, and simply lack the necessary knowledge or resources to prepare a satisfactory proposal. But it is also possible that such assistance acts as a distortion of priorities. Since comparable support for preparing other requests is less readily available. To quote Muraskin (2004, p. 1923): 'The GAVI was designed for the countries' good but not by the countries. It is vital to realize that the demand for this initiative did not emanate from the designated beneficiaries. Rather, the countries as a group have had to be wooed, "educated," and financially enticed to accept the GAVI's goals as their own'.

The dilemma is well illustrated by the case of health systems. There has been much debate in connection with GAVI as to whether the Alliance should place more emphasis on health system support, which is perhaps the most obvious example of a 'horizontal' as opposed to 'vertical' initiative. Some, especially several European countries, argued that GAVI should not focus so single-mindedly on vaccines but should also finance health systems strengthening (HSS), and a study commissioned by the GAVI Board recommended that the Alliance consider strengthening health systems as part of an 'enhanced effort' to help those countries falling behind in their immunisation coverage targets (McKinsey and Company 2003, quoted in Naimoli 2009). Despite some resistance (including, reportedly, from Bill Gates) this view gained support, and GAVI has in recent years made a major strategic shift, allocating substantial sums also to HSS. 'Because of the generous funding made available by the IFFI donors, the GAVI investment in HSS is sizable. In early 2008, the GAVI Board added US$300 million to the original US$500 million allocation, for a total investment of US$800 million' (Naimoli 2009, p. 8). Naimoli gives credit to GAVI for having taken 'a bold step in trying to carry through on the longstanding challenge in global health to bridge the divide between vertical and horizontal modes of delivering priority health services' (Naimoli 2009, p. 19). But he notes also the risk that this entails—well recognised also by GAVI: 'from the outset, the GAVI Board acknowledged that HSS represented a significant risk for the Alliance' (GAVI 2005, p. 12, quoted in Naimoli 2009). The original strategy, of focusing on immunisation, is clearly a much safer option.

It is not difficult to understand why a vertical, top-down initiative with a focus on immunisation is so attractive to the donor community. Other measures to improve health, such as HSS, are more difficult to implement and more difficult to justify in terms of the rather narrow economic logic of international donors; it is also more difficult to demonstrate that they have achieved concrete results. These arguments are not so different from those advanced by Walsh and Warren in 1979.

Opinions regarding the merits of including HSS in GAVI were very mixed. Some of the main countervailing arguments were as follows:

> Evidence for proven, cost-effective, system-targeted interventions for overcoming documented barriers not presented; investment viewed as a 'leap of faith'. . . .
>
> Improving outcomes beyond immunization may be too complex and ambitious for a vaccine-preventable disease partnership with little experience in broader maternal-child health programming or health systems development. . . . Poorer countries should not receive more money because of absorptive and management capacity concerns. (Naimoli 2009, pp. 9–10)

Based on substantial empirical evidence, Naimoli (2009) assesses the initial results of the HSS component of GAVI and shows that there have been problems of precisely the kind that were anticipated. HSS is indeed difficult to implement. But the argument concerning national capacity is problematic. The conclusion can readily be drawn that those countries that most need assistance should not get it. 'Absorptive capacity' is one of the most basic problems that have beset development assistance since it first began: the countries that most urgently need assistance are precisely those which are least able to make effective use of it (see, for example, McNeill 1981). A disturbing paradox arises in which pressure to spend money confronts countries in great need, but with limited capacity to use it well. The bureaucracy in a poor country, overburdened at the top level, accepts technical assistance for planning and implementation, thus relying on consultants and donors to prepare proposals and, in effect, allowing them a substantial impact on priority-setting. To quote Naimoli's rather cautious wording: 'there are questions about the degree to which the government has exercised sufficient control over the identification of its assistance needs' (Naimoli 2009, p. 18).

Today, more than ever, GAVI (and donors in general) require 'evidence' in quantitative form in order to justify their expenditure. The danger is not only that global actors risk sidelining the governments of weaker countries in setting priorities, they may also ignore the information that is provided by governments, replacing it with their own. A recent analysis suggests that 'evidence to support health systems strengthening strategies is still extremely weak' (Bosch-Capblanch et al. 2011). But the same study also finds that governments' own data are hardly used. 'Nation-wide household surveys were scarcely cited in the health systems strengthening proposals even though they provide data not only on immunization coverage but also on household and system characteristics that may be related to the uptake of vaccination.' '(W)e found that in 39 of the

44 countries that submitted proposals there had been nation-wide household surveys (DHS or MICS) that could have been used to support descriptions of the immunisation status of the population and/or specific barriers to immunisation. However, only 12 of those 39 countries (31%) used survey findings to support their requests.' (Bosch-Capblanch et al. 2011)

Donors' demand for statistics is perhaps even greater when it comes to measuring performance *ex post*, seeking to show that targets have been achieved. Donors' obsession with targets has increased further as a result of the Millennium Development Goals. This in turn led to a fixation on (often unreliable) statistics, as one very well-informed commentator has noted: 'Statistics have been abused to fabricate evidence of success. The great paradox is that poverty is increasingly regarded as a multi-dimensional phenomenon whilst its quantification remains essentially one-dimensional, which reinforces a money-metric perspective of the MDGs. The agenda has been cut back to a standard set of macroeconomic, sectoral or institutional reforms of a technical nature' (Vandemoortele 2011, p. 1). 'The MDGs have been distorted and misconstrued as objectives that can be reached through technical interventions funded by foreign aid to scale up investments and replicate lessons learnt elsewhere' (Vandemoortele 2011, p. 18). Immunisation is a good example of precisely this.

The setting of targets is closely linked to the increasing pressure from donor countries for aid in all sectors to be results-based, justified in terms of 'development effectiveness'. This follows a period in which recipient countries were termed 'partners' and aid was increasingly given to budget support, implying more freedom to the recipient country and less demand for performance accountability. The increasing emphasis on measurement of performance relates not just to outputs, but also outcomes and impacts—all to be based on objective indicators. One of the attractions of immunisation is precisely its measurability: both as regards specifying targets and measuring achievement. The 'target group' can, at least in principle, be accurately quantified: the total number of children in a certain age group. (This is often simply, but rather misleadingly, equated with 'demand'). The standard output–outcome–impact evaluation procedure thus appears relatively easy to apply. The output is X million vaccines delivered. The outcome is Y million children protected (the link from output to outcome being here quite strong, provided—and this is important—that vaccines are correctly administered and that there is no wastage). The impact is Z number of lives saved. As noted in Chapter 1, setting and achieving numerical targets is essential for mobilising and sustaining financial support for vaccination. Donors, not least GAVI, need to be convinced that their money is well spent; that the funding has led to real achievements. But whose numbers are judged reliable, and by whom? Statistics may be collected by different actors, both national and global, and perhaps for different purposes. The above account of the NUVI retreat exemplifies concern about how burden of disease figures may be used or misused. The situation is further complicated by the fact that some of those involved seem to be so committed to the cause that they regard numbers as a means to an end—advocacy of vaccines—rather than a basis for objectively assessing the merits of alternative priority setting (Muraskin 2004).

And this brings the discussion back to the central issue of accountability. At issue is not just the extent to which GAVI is accountable by comparison, say, with an international organisation such as the WHO, and the annual WHA. The more general, and more important, issue is the extent to which global actors in the immunisation field are accountable to poor people in poor countries—the 'recipients'—as opposed to the donors. William Muraskin has called for the 'inverted pyramid of the GAVI' to be turned on its head. 'Top-down globalism', he writes, 'plays a necessary and powerful role in initially moving the public health community forward, but it cannot succeed in the long run without genuine bottom-up input and support' (Muraskin 2004, p. 1922).

Conclusions

The power and authority of the many different actors that make up the immunisation system vary considerably, and as a result relations between them are generally unequal. Money is, as it long has been, a very important source of power in this system. The volume of global funding—both for health in general and for immunisation in particular—has increased considerably in the last two decades, with the BMGF playing a crucial role. This has had an impact both on horizontal relations between global actors and on vertical relations between global actors and national governments. The system may be seen as a pyramid—from the global through the national to the local—in which money is a major source of power and authority, exercised by global actors at the 'top'. Those who receive money are required to account for their actions to those who grant it—reporting on performance and results.

Although it has come to dominate, money is not the only source of authority in the global immunisation system. Expertise is another. And whilst it too is largely exercised by actors at 'the top', expertise can more easily be challenged, at least where counter expertise is available. (In Chapter 4 we will present an instance of this.) As shown in this chapter, global actors in the vaccination field have often had differing, and to some extent even conflicting, priorities. On some occasions these actors have tended to coordinate and cooperate, on others to engage in conflict and competition. Moreover the structure of the global level, with which this chapter has been concerned, the overall configuration of actors, is not fixed. Since 1999 GAVI has not only made massive financial contributions, but also brought an increasing degree of unity, coordination, and coherence to the sector. A consequence of this, however, has been a growing influence by global actors, and especially GAVI, over national policy-making.

Chapter 4

National commitments and global objectives

Kristin Sandberg and Judith Justice

Introduction

The success or failure of global immunisation efforts depends on how initiatives and policies translate into programmes at the country level. It is striking that national immunisation programmes are expected to function in an identical manner that is structured by the logistics of a cold chain designed to ensure the safe and effective transmission of technology from manufacturer to health clinics. This uniform model of national immunisation programme functioning stands in contrast to the vast and clearly apparent differences among countries, most notably their political systems and levels of economic development. The well-documented variations in the ability of countries to organise health provision for their populations might be expected to explain variations in how well immunisation programmes work in reality. Yet, as our studies from Malawi and India show, this does not appear to be the case. And in fragile states such as Sierra Leone and Afghanistan, child immunisation programmes have been held up as one health intervention that works.

   As the historical account in Chapter 1 showed, the expansion of national immunisation programmes embodied in the EPI was the result of careful and gradual encouragement of national authorities by WHO and UNICEF. From a global perspective, it makes sense to encourage all countries to participate in a concerted effort to control infectious disease, as the full benefits can only be reaped if all participate and no delinquent country or region remains as a source for transmission. This 'global herd immunity', it has been argued, can be viewed as a global public good and a justification for eradication initiatives, first of smallpox and subsequently of polio (Barrett 2007). This rather technical viewpoint is complemented by the moral perspective that figured prominently during the formation of the GAVI Alliance: if a vaccine is available on the international market, to not make it available to all children, particularly those whose poverty makes them most vulnerable, is a form of moral neglect on the part of the international community (Sandberg et al. 2010).

The combined rationale—both technical and moral—inspired the global immunisation effort to reach populations worldwide. However, between global immunisation efforts and target populations stand national governments. The sovereignty of nation states, the right to decide over their own territories and populations, is a fundamental principle of the international community, to be breached only under extreme circumstances. The cooperation of national governments is required if global immunisation initiatives are to reach people on a nationwide scale, both as a matter of principle, but also—to varying extents—in practice. The variation in extent is dependent on the relative power of global actors and national governments. This chapter looks at the global–national interface: the places where global and national actors involved with immunisation meet each other. It elucidates the political processes that shape country responses to, and their implementation of, global policies and goals. The variety of such interfaces is a consequence of the wide range of global initiatives (including the Polio Eradication Initiative and the Measles Vaccine Initiative), as well as the various ways in which technical assistance relating to routine immunisation services are provided by international organisations, donors, NGOs, and international research institutions. Within the immunisation field, we focus especially on the issue of new vaccine introduction, using it as a probe, allowing for an in-depth account of the interactions that shape implementation.

In order to capture the diversity of interactions between the global and national levels, the chapter draws on a growing literature on new vaccine introduction, as well as on research we carried out in Malawi and India. These cases bring to the fore the question of national ownership of policy-making on immunisation. We also explore changes in the relations between global initiatives and national governments that have paralleled the rise of new vaccine introduction on the global immunisation agenda over the past decade. We address questions such as: Under what conditions do countries agree to introduce new vaccines? To what extent and under what conditions does resistance to global actors emerge, and what forms does it take? Are funds refused, recommended new vaccines not taken up, or global priorities or authority challenged?

We start by mapping the meeting places between global and national actors at the country level regarding immunisation: the sites at which global and national decision-makers interact. What types of actors are involved, and with what roles and interests? The chapter subsequently makes use of ideas from political science and health policy analysis to put into perspective what is known about the process and dynamics of the global–national interaction on new vaccines. On the basis of these observations, we argue that the manner in which vaccine

introductions unfold remains a political process that reflects the quirks and pecu-
liarities of each individual country. Recognising the significance of the national
political dimension then leads us to pose the question: What are the national perspectives on immunisation, and how do they interact with the global view?

Immunisation at the interface of the global and the national

Meeting places between global and national institutions concerned with public
health date back to colonial times. We can think of the missionary health services, the institutes of tropical medicine that were established under colonial
auspices and of the work of philanthropic foundations (including the Rockefeller Foundation) in the same period. In the course of the last half century the
United Nations system and its specialist organisations have of course come to
play a prominent role. In the last two decades the pattern has evolved further
with the rise of global health initiatives, some of which have become key links
between global and country actors working to improve health. One important
interface site is the regional and country offices of key global actors, where global and national representatives frequently meet. Other sites may be less apparent, perhaps emerging as a result of broad changes in the nature of international
engagement. Where precisely should we look, in relation to immunisation?

Consider the application process by which countries request support from
the GAVI Alliance. When GAVI was formed in 2000, only countries with a
gross national income per capita below US$1000 could apply. Beginning in
2011, the ceiling was raised to US$1500 (based on World Bank data), with some
flexibilities so that countries graduating from the lower-income brackets could
be considered for continued support, as could countries with large birth
cohorts, such as India (and earlier also China and Indonesia). As of 2012, the
main types of support countries apply for are 'new and underused vaccines' and
health systems strengthening. Support for new vaccine introduction represents
by far the largest share of disbursements, with US$506 million compared to
US$78 million for health systems, according to the 2010 Annual Financial
Report (GAVI 2010). According to the same source, new vaccine support
increased by 237% from 2006 to 2010. Thus it is the poorest countries that are
favoured by GAVI, together with emerging economies with large populations
(not least because of the contribution these can make to the achievement of
MDG4). It is here that global–national relations may have the most powerful
influence on immunisation.

When GAVI was created, a notable feature was that the Alliance would not
have its own country representation, but was designed to work through its

partners, the most important at country level being WHO and UNICEF. WHO has a strong standing as the main technical advisor on health for all through its regional and its country offices. WHO country offices are often located close to MoHs and play a key advisory role on immunisation issues. UNICEF has a complementary role, taking responsibility for shipments, logistics, and cold-chain management. In addition, countries with very weak health systems, or in crisis, also receive support from UNICEF for running immunisation services as part of health clinics, often in collaboration with local and international NGOs.

National stakeholders may include, in addition to MoHs and EPI managers, professional bodies, institutes of medical research, and national paediatric societies. Donor countries also play a role through their diplomatic representation, as traditional bilateral supporters of the EPI. As we will see later in the chapter, the increased demand for scientific evidence in decision-making processes relating to new vaccine introduction has also brought international scientific experts (e.g. from the Center for Disease Control in Atlanta or the Johns Hopkins University) to the decision-making table.

As part of the Polio Eradication Initiative, governments and national WHO offices established platforms known as Interagency Coordination Committees (ICCs) to facilitate coordination of all actors involved with immunisation at the country level; a good example of an interface site. When GAVI was established, these ICCs were expanded to address issues of monitoring and implementation of GAVI support. The existence of such a committee became a key prerequisite for submitting a GAVI application (Grundy 2010, p. 187). The number and constellation of actors involved, and the ways they collaborate in the ICCs in planning and preparing applications to GAVI, differ among countries. In the initial phase of GAVI, an independent study by the London School of Hygiene and Tropical Medicine and Save the Children UK reviewed the first application process from a country perspective (Starling et al. 2002). All four subSaharan countries in the study (Mozambique, Tanzania, Ghana, and Lesotho) had already established ICCs. They functioned as planning units for National Immunization Days of the Polio Eradication Campaign as well as for measles immunisation campaigns and neonatal tetanus control. What they also had in common was that all were chaired by the MoH, with the EPI manager as secretary, and WHO and UNICEF as regular attendees. In Tanzania and Mozambique, World Bank representatives also attended, as did the EU and the United Nations Population Fund (UNFPA) in Mozambique. In all countries, bilateral aid agencies in different constellations and the civil society organisation Rotary were also involved. Only in Ghana, among the four countries, was there any representation from national professional organisations (the Paediatric Society of Ghana and the

Institute for Medical Research). The study found that despite their formally similar structures, the actual functioning of these ICCs varied, depending on working relationships between the various participants: government, international agencies, and bilateral donors. The authority of the different actors in the ICCs would vary significantly depending on their relative power—derived from financial resources, mandate, technical expertise etc.

This early study of the application process, which is one of only a few independent studies of GAVI overall, observed that links between country authorities and GAVI were largely indirect, mediated by multilateral members of the ICC, or by the visiting international consultants or experts who helped prepare the application. All countries received this kind of external technical support '... either directly from GAVI or arranged and funded by it' (Starling et al. 2002, p. 23). Such support is needed because of the newness and speed of the application process. Another point of contact was through the international workshops and meetings organised by the WHO Regional Office for Africa or by GAVI directly. Although national MoHs in principle steered the overall application process, this was not always what happened in practice, as we shall see presently.

The discussions on Financial Sustainability Plans that followed the first round of applications to GAVI provided an important site for contact between global and national actors. Work on this topic was intended to create a shared understanding of what sustainability meant in the context of low-income countries with rising immunisation budgets. It was also intended to assist in developing productive relations between ministries of finance and of health. In June 2001, the GAVI Alliance partners reached a definition for 'sustainable financing', as '... a shared responsibility of both governments and their development partners' (Milstien et al. 2008, p. 6701). A task force under the GAVI secretariat, the Financing Task Force, developed a model for helping countries develop Financial Sustainability Plans. In the spirit of the Alliance this would be done through an approach of 'multi-partner implementation', (Milstien et al. 2008, p. 6702). In practice, this apparently meant financing of 'capacity-building activities' in individual countries, supported by key GAVI partners, such as WHO, UNICEF, and the World Bank, through central donors such as the Norwegian, British or American aid agencies (NORAD, DfID, and USAID, respectively) or through international organisations, for example PATH and the Agence de Médicine Préventive (AMP). It can be argued that—at least in the poorest countries—the initial concept of GAVI, as an alliance, enhanced the involvement of multiple global actors, with their considerable power and authority.

In 2006, the BMGF commissioned a scoping study to explore a closely related issue: to develop capacity at the country level that would assist national stakeholders in determining '... whether, when and how to adopt innovations in immunisation programmes' (Druce et al. 2006, p. 5). The study placed a major emphasis on evidence, and among the observations was that low-, middle-, and high-income countries have in common that decision-making tended to be ad hoc and informal, with limited capacity in MoHs '... to commission, review and analyze evidence'. There was a need for more *informed* and *transparent* decision-making processes (Druce et al. 2006, pp. 6–7, emphasis added). The resulting Supporting Independent Immunization Vaccine and Advisory Committees Initiative was funded and initiated in 2008. AMP and the International Vaccine Institute in Seoul, Korea, in collaboration with WHO, are key stakeholders. Other partners include UNICEF, GAVI, PATH, and the CDC. The initiative works to support middle-income countries and countries eligible for GAVI support in the establishment or strengthening of National Technical Advisory Groups for Immunization (NTAGI) (Senouci et al. 2010). In a recent survey conducted by the Initiative, 61% of 147 responding countries reported to have an Advisory Group in place (Bryson et al. 2010).

In a review of 15 National Technical Advisory Groups across all country income levels, it was found that the majority of participants are national, and that the MoH plays a central role as chair or secretary. Members have scientific expertise primarily in vaccinology, medicine, and public health, and less often in economics. In some cases committees have consumer or community 'lay' representatives (Gessner et al. 2010). Most committees also include non-voting members, such as the EPI leadership, regulatory offices or government vaccine producers, or representatives from organisations such as UNICEF or WHO. (The pharmaceutical industry rarely participate as members, but could be called upon to present information.) The legal responsibilities of the groups vary among countries, although in most cases they were set up to advise government decision-makers.

More and more new vaccines are becoming available, and some of them (initially at least) are very expensive. Faced with deciding which should be introduced into national immunisation programmes, a standard set of criteria—disease burden, the safety and effectiveness of the vaccine, the cost-effectiveness of vaccination, and so on—appeals to policy-makers, even in rich countries (Vyse et al. 2002; Gezondheidsraad 2007; Smith et al. 2009). Applying such criteria in practice, however, depends on evidence: on the availability of reliable epidemiological, scientific, and economic data. In its advocacy work the GAVI Alliance (and the global health community more generally, as well, of course, as the vaccine industry) has stressed that vaccines as tools to save lives should be made available to all those who need them. How are decisions on their introduction made at country level? The available literature gives the impression of initial high involvement of global actors in the early phases of the GAVI Alliance when the process was new, but increased emphasis on country ownership—a much debated concept—with the heightened need for prioritisation among new vaccines. In order to understand how global perspectives are introduced to and negotiated at the national level, we need to examine how such processes actually function in practice.

Standing back: how do countries and the international community interact?

When countries engage in decision-making processes on immunisation and new vaccines, they do so within a context of multiple parallel interactions with global actors, involving a range of global health initiatives, all of which are trying to have their particular schemes and priorities implemented. To help us understand how the national and global domains interact, we can draw on some broader ideas in the field of international relations, where scholars have addressed the growing salience of global governance and global public policy and its consequences for individual countries.

The global policy domain has expanded its influence since the 1990s, introducing '. . . opportunities for and constraints upon both global and national governance that did not exist in the past' (Ruggie 2004, p. 504). This domain is a result of broader historical developments, and defined as '. . . an increasingly institutionalized transnational arena of discourse, contestation, and action concerning the production of global public goods, involving private as well as public actors' (Ruggie 2004, p. 504). Global public policy is more than the sum of cooperation between nation states. A new feature of the global domain, exemplified by the change in IHR adopted in 2005, is that it not only addresses issues and interests that states bring to the decision-making tables, but also those raised by non-state actors like civil society or industry (Kaul 2006). Nevertheless, and importantly, it is national governments that implement global policies. The increasing pressure on states to respond to global expectations has led some to speak of 'the intermediary state', where states no longer have exclusive authority over domestic policy-making, but rather find themselves in a position of having to blend external and domestic policy demands, thus blurring global and national decision-making (Kaul 2006).

The instruments of implementation and enforcement available in the global domain are limited. Money is certainly a powerful instrument in poor countries, while the promotion of norms is more important elsewhere. Policy visions and demands can be conceptualised as expectations transmitted through intergovernmental forums, international business, civil society organisations, global media, and multiactor venues like the World Economic Forum, which in fact was the venue for the launch of the GAVI Alliance in 1999. Thus, as development expert Inge Kaul argues, '. . . international public policy-making is an increasingly busy process, with multiple actors heaping layer upon layer on to the global stockpile of policy norms and, most important, expecting in ever more demanding terms, that states will accept them as guideposts of national policymaking' (Kaul 2006).

How do states respond to increasing global policy expectations? A comparative case study of 19 low- and higher-income countries focusing on the roles of states in relation to the international policy-making domain in general found a significant difference among countries (Kaul 2006). High-income countries tended to view international cooperation as an 'outgoing' process: one on which they could exert influence. Their response to incoming policy demands was limited. For the lowest income countries, the opposite was true. Thus international cooperation within national borders is more common in some states than others, being particularly common in low-income countries. For many low-income countries, Kaul suggests, rejecting international interference is not an option, since it carries the risk of losing the support on which they rely; they are obliged to be responsive to global policies.

Still, while international relations scholars emphasise that the aim of global policies is to enhance global welfare, health policy scholars remind us that the top-down model of implementation endorses authority and control being exercised from above (Erasmus and Gilson 2008). One may then challenge a situation in which the global domain determines policy objectives, which countries are then required merely to implement. Might a more 'bottom-up' view, a country perspective, lead one to question the appropriateness of global public policy goals in a given country setting? What about the discretionary power of state agents, responsible for implementation at the country level? Implementation work depends so much on local political and social circumstances: complexities over which global decision-makers can hardly have a full overview. In this way, whilst global actors may strive for conformity, countries may wish to preserve some discretion in implementation. Erasmus and Gilson argue that such discretion is a form of informal authority. It may be frowned upon by higher-level policy-making agents, but can be essential in the adaptation of policies to local circumstances. What may be seen 'from the top' as resistance or subversion might well be a country adapting to their own circumstances a policy that they fully support.

Within the relatively new discourse on global policies the field of immunisation offers an interesting example, since the global domain has here been a prevailing force for many decades. Global immunisation policies have appeared justified by the need for technical streamlining, for coordination, and to ensure efficacy and safety of vaccines. As we saw earlier, the dominant interpretation of the global smallpox eradication campaign was to the effect that country conformity leads to national as well as global welfare gains. Thereafter, the UCI campaign of the 1990s reiterated the need to ensure that national governments responded to the goals set out by the global campaign. The goals of the campaign appeared self-evident; what might be needed (in addition to funding) was national commitment. Some key global actors saw it as their task to bring this about; in a tribute to UNICEF leader Jim Grant, the idea of creating political will in countries is central:

'How many late night conversations have ended with the words *"you can't do anything without political will."* How many plans and potentials have come to nothing for the lack of this political will? Jim Grant's response was: *"Well, we'll just have to create the political will.""* (Adamson 2001, p. 26)

In practice, political will has often entailed the identification of a national champion, a president or a first lady who would make immunisation their special cause. Undoubtedly, a cause that is high on the global agenda generates its own incentives for such a national champion to take it up. However, as the global health agenda grows more complex, so must national responses become more sophisticated. Political will is no longer sufficient for solving the implementation puzzle at the national level. Although it remains important, capacity for implementation and actual coordination undoubtedly also play a role. Increasingly, this capacity relates not just to the ability to shift vaccines from warehouse to clinic, but to achieving transparency and accountability in multi-actor decision-making processes. In this way, nation states retain a key role, with clear rights to self-determination enshrined in the principle of sovereignty. In addition, among the principles of the Constitution of WHO are government responsibility for '. . . the health of their peoples which can be fulfilled only by the provision of adequate health and social measures' (p. 1).

The country perspective: new vaccine adoption

National decision-making on the adoption of new vaccines has received increased attention since 2005, both from policy actors such as the WHO and GAVI, and from the research community at large. This has been partly due to the increase in the number of new vaccines reaching the market. In the context of global health, a crucial and distinctive point about vaccines is that—unlike curative medicine—the demand does not, generally, arise from the people themselves. (In the event of a sudden disease outbreak the situation may be different). In this way, government constitutes the source of demand and the key link between global efforts and populations. What Horton and Das (2011, p. 296) call 'the vaccine paradox' is that governments are the main agents both of demand and provision, negotiating 'terms of engagement' with the population. It is interesting to study how they perform this role, of linking global efforts with actual outcomes.

Instead of demand from their people, governments (at least those of poor countries) respond to policies and support from the global domain. Global policies and norms sometimes take the form of pressure, manifested explicitly in targets such as MDG4, backed up by evidence. The evidence typically consists of a combination of scientific, epidemiological, and economic information, which can provide the basis for deciding whether or not to introduce a new vaccine. If the need for governments to choose among several new vaccines is relatively recent, what was the situation in the late 1990s prior to GAVI's establishment? A study commissioned by the CVI in 1999 found that local evidence and the fit with national needs and priorities (including competing priorities within the health sector) played an important role for countries when considering adopting new vaccines (Justice 2000b). Neither WHO nor UNICEF was actively promoting new vaccines in a situation where many countries, particularly in Africa, were recognised as having weak, even dysfunctional, delivery systems. Under such conditions, new vaccine introduction could threaten to be a major disruption, and the focus was on strengthening the EPI, replacing deteriorating cold chains, and ensuring financial sustainability for the six basic vaccines included in routine immunisation. It was notable, however, that the chances of a new vaccine being taken into consideration were higher in certain situations: where countries were host to major vaccine trials, if international donors played a particular advocacy role, or if senior political figures or heads of state were champions of a particular new vaccine, (Justice 2000b). Nevertheless, the majority of countries introducing new vaccines in the 1990s were high- and middle-income countries.

Since the creation of GAVI, a major change is that thanks to GAVI support the poorest countries are introducing new vaccines faster than many middle-income countries (Makinen et al. 2012; Shearer et al. 2010). While all countries depend on WHO for normative standards and technical advice, there is a division among countries, for instance depending on their eligibility for receiving GAVI assistance such as income level, described above. As we shall see below when examining how the decision-making process plays out in reality, the global health community and particularly donor agencies can have a strong influence on vaccine adoption. In this way, donor countries are prominent policy-makers in the global domain on immunisation issues, while recipients of assistance feature largely as policy-takers.

Before referring specifically to Malawi and India, we first turn to the growing body of publications on national decision-making processes on new vaccine introduction. A systematic review of the literature on national decision-making on adopting new vaccines found that roughly a third of the papers presented frameworks for decision-making, putting forward distinctly normative policy prescriptions. Such papers focus on what countries ought to consider when going through a decision-making process (Burchett et al. 2012). (Only a fifth of these papers were published prior to 2004, demonstrating how interest in decision-making processes intensified in response to GAVI activities). Out of the criteria included in each of the 21 proposed frameworks, the most frequently listed were burden of disease information, vaccine efficacy, effectiveness and safety, programmatic considerations of feasibility, public acceptability of the vaccine, and economic evaluations (Burchett et al. 2012, e.g. Mansoor et al. 2000; Mahoney 2004; Munira and Fritzen 2007). But in practice, decision-making processes are far less technical endeavours. They typically involve a mix of political, financial, logistical, and scientific considerations, and the interplay of various interests. The expanding *empirical* literature on vaccine introduction contrasts with the normative literature and reveals that decision-making processes are indeed rather complex. A comparative case study of seven low- and middle-income countries concluded that decisions to introduce new vaccines are first and foremost shaped by domestic politics. Real-life decisions in the countries studied bore little resemblance to the decision-making frameworks devised to guide vaccine introduction (Burchett et al. 2012). Studies of real-life decisions are what is needed to contribute to an understanding of how vaccines are introduced in practice.

Prior to the GAVI Alliance, the only new vaccine available to low-income countries was the hepatitis B vaccine; with the Hib vaccine slowly coming on board as a vaccine whose introduction GAVI would support (Justice 2000b). A few years later a pertinent choice for governments introducing vaccines with GAVI support was whether to add new antigens as single vaccines, or in quadri- or pentavalent combination vaccines, considered in relation to logistics and possible needs to revise cold-chain and storage requirements, but where final decisions were often influenced by availability from manufacturers.

In the first phase of GAVI, the concern with decision-making processes also addressed the role of donor agencies at country level. It was noted that in countries where coordination mechanisms were driven by a small number of donors, there was a risk of foregoing the opportunity of building country capacity. Yet it appears that this was what happened in, for instance, Mozambique, where bilateral donors involved in the initial introduction of new vaccines were reported as highly critical of the process, adding yet another global health initiative to the government's agenda (Brugha et al. 2002). A study of decision-making in GAVI-recipient countries commissioned by the BMGF concluded that '. . . decisions are driven less by national technical considerations, than by national and international political and financial factors. Global and national disease champions, including external technical agencies, tend to be major drivers of the decision-making process' (Druce et al. 2006, p. 11). Moreover, the study continues, '. . . technical and donor agencies have major and sometimes disproportionate influence on national decisions', explained by the best funded programmes tending to be more vocal at the national level (Druce et al. 2006).

In brief, the early experience in GAVI recipient countries was that decision-making processes tended to be programme driven (e.g. GAVI Alliance) and disease specific (e.g. advocates for the hepatitis B vaccines or against Japanese encephalitis), and stakeholders argued that a more evidence-informed process was required, anchored more broadly in health systems planning, to ensure that evidence across alternative interventions could be compared. If countries did not have adequate disease surveillance systems or scientific capacity to carry out studies, global actors would step in to assist. The implication is that when low- and middle-income countries introduce new vaccines as a response to global health initiatives, donors and technical agencies (GAVI, WHO, UNICEF) are becoming stakeholders in national decision-making processes. As an illustration, starting in 2001 GAVI offered to assist in the introduction of Hib vaccine. However, it soon became clear that Hib-vaccine introduction was lagging behind expectations in most GAVI-eligible countries. In 2005 GAVI therefore established the Hib Initiative in the form of a consortium based at the Johns Hopkins University in the USA, and also including the London School of Hygiene and Tropical Medicine, WHO and the CDC. Its role involved helping governments clarify whether they should adopt the Hib-containing pentavalent vaccine, based on evaluation of scientific evidence of need and on advocacy. The initiative saw its task as to 'build political will', by expanding the group of stakeholders, customising information material, and getting passionate people to speak up for the introduction of Hib vaccine. Advocacy arenas are regional and national meetings which convene policy-makers, paediatricians, and policy-makers. From the Hib Initiative's perspective, linking GAVI objectives with MDGs has been a very effective advocacy strategy; after establishment of the Initiative, the share of eligible countries introducing the vaccine rose from 25% in 2006 to 46% in 2010 (Zuber et al. 2011).

The demand that decision-making be evidence-based, or at least evidence-informed, is well established for high-income countries (though the weight to be attached to various kinds of evidence might be disputed). On the other hand, it is rather recent for many low-income countries. Evidence here relates primarily to the burden of a disease against which a vaccine will protect. Ideally, such information also includes an economic analysis to determine the cost-effectiveness of introduction. Disease burden data often reveal substantial differences between countries and regions; while some preventable infectious diseases are common for most countries, such as diphtheria, tetanus or a childhood illness like measles, others are more bound to geographic regions, like Japanese enchephalitis and tuberculosis. Some, like pneumococcal disease and rotavirus, may occur universally but be far more serious in areas of poverty.

Is evidence used? In the case of the introduction of the pentavalent vaccine, a concern within WHO, among development partners and within the academic community, is that evidence is not properly used in determining policy (Druce et al. 2006, p. 14). This study, based on inquiries in Bangladesh, Uganda, and Senegal, reports limited involvement by researchers and other members of civil society in the policy process. It found further that when burden of disease data are included in the studies, they tended to have been commissioned by external agencies. A further problem, which we shall return to below, was that disease prevalence data were often not connected to any assessment of the cost-benefit of introduction. More recent studies underline the difficulty of generating the local burden of disease data. Scott Jordon et al. (2012) refer to immunisation experts in WHO regional offices who claim that only 23% of low- and lower-middle-income countries have published estimates of Hib meningitis incidence and call for a greater willingness by countries to accept regional data as proxies. The absence of local data exacerbates the problem of external pressure for introduction. Research suggests that lower-middle-income countries, many of which are not eligible for GAVI support, consider it 'essential' to have country-specific data when deciding to introduce new vaccines; burden of disease data from neighbouring countries is considered less valuable (Makinen et al. 2012).

The case for introducing a new vaccine is ultimately tied to capacity to pay. Cost-effectiveness evaluation is one of the basic tools of policy evaluation, which is meant to demonstrate whether or not the expected health- or societal gains justify the expenditure entailed. But feasibility in social cost-benefit terms is different from the question of financial sustainability—a problem which is well known in development aid: will government or donors be able to finance the vaccine into the future? Studies covering the early GAVI Alliance years noted a lack of analysis both of cost-effectiveness and of long-term financial feasibility. From an independent and critical viewpoint decision-making could be described as '. . . essentially a supply-driven process', affecting the adoption of '. . . potentially unsustainable new commodities' (Brugha et al. 2002, p. 437). At the same time it has been suggested that from the perspective of countries eligible for GAVI support sustainability may not be seen as an issue, in view of the availability of external earmarked funding (Druce et al. 2006, p. 20). The scoping study mentioned earlier on evidence-based decisions found that new vaccine introduction was not discussed as part of the sector-wide approach in the countries surveyed. Moreover, information on cost and cost implications was rarely asked for by government; uncertainty about future vaccine prices was often used as an argument in favour of adoption, expecting that increasing markets would be a key factor in eventually bringing down prices (Druce et al. 2006.).

However, the presence of external funding is not necessarily a guarantee that costs will be taken care of; changes in aid instruments, vaccine prices, and even the eligibility status of a country for support can all affect the situation. For example, a review of lessons learned for GAVI in its first phase from 2000 to 2005 observed that changing behaviours of donor countries were adding to concerns about financial sustainability, as donors who were either contributing to the sector-wide approach (SWAp) or who had made a large-scale commitment to GAVI at the global level were ceasing to earmark funding for immunisation at the country level. The rationalisation by donors that their contribution at the global level would suffice challenged '. . . the assumption that GAVI acts as a "lever" for increased donor support for immunisation at the country level' (HLSP 2005, p. 20). Country stakeholders at a New and Underused Vaccines Implementation (NUVI) workshop placed the issue of financial sustainability in a dynamic perspective, reflecting on previous gaps in GAVI funding and previous experiences with fluctuations in long-term donor funding, and voicing a concern for immunisation financing in the medium and long term (Scott Jordon et al. 2012). As noted also in Chapter 3, referring to another NUVI meeting, this is a touchy issue. Countries whose GNP per capita rises, and which thereby lose their eligibility for GAVI support, face a dilemma, even given provisions for transitional support. The extent to which it worries countries highlights the magnitude of the financial commitment that introduction of a new vaccine represents.

Some countries have a domestic vaccine industry catering principally to the national market. This can have significant implications. Thus a study of new vaccine adoption in Indonesia and China, which both have a domestic manufacturing base, did not find price to be an important factor for introduction (Makinen et al. 2012). Having a domestic vaccine industry, however, can also make government decision-making processes more complex as industrial interests with regards to specific vaccines interlink health and immunisation policy-making with policies of biotechnology and trade.

It is notable that studies on country decision-making on immunisation concentrate solely on new vaccine introduction and have little to say regarding routine immunisation issues or health systems concerns. This could be a bias in the literature, but may also imply that vaccine introduction processes tend to be narrowly focused on new vaccines themselves, without considering the costs and implications of new vaccine introduction for national immunisation systems, including training of personnel, cold-chain expansion, and revised immunisation schedules (Scott Jordon et al. 2012).

Is the situation different for high-income countries? The literature suggests that factors weigh differently across countries, with public perceptions considered of higher importance for decision-making in high-income countries, while issues related to programmatic feasibility and affordability are more important for other countries (Burchett et al. 2012). Increasingly, however, all countries face the similar challenge of introducing multiple new vaccines, whether simultaneously or sequentially (see, for example, Scott Jordon et al. 2012).

The systematic review of the vaccine introduction literature we discussed earlier notes that the normative frameworks put forward in some publications pay no attention to the criteria that are actually important in one country or another. They lack any detailed explorations of actual policy-making processes (Burchett et al. 2011). We turn now to an in-depth examination of *how* the decision-making process actually unfolds in two very different countries, India and Malawi.

Malawi: a 'model country'

Malawi presents an interesting case for studying key factors influencing differential immunisation coverage and the introduction of new vaccines since despite its weak economy and under-resourced health system, it is among the early adopters of new vaccines (Nyirenda and Justice, 2012).

Malawi is a small country (15.2 million inhabitants) located in Southern Africa. On the Human Development Index it ranks as one of the poorest countries in the world. Despite its poverty and the challenges posed by a high rate of HIV/AIDS infection (12%), high rates of maternal mortality and child malnutrition, and a chronic shortage of health workers, Malawi has high immunisation coverage (approximately 92%), is among the early adopters of new vaccines, and is expected to reduce child mortality sufficiently to achieve MDG4 by 2015. Malawi is an aid-dependent country, with 60% of total health expenditure coming from external sources (WHO 2009c). As a result, representatives of donor organisations and members of the global health community tend to be active participants in decision-making processes related to health and immunisation.

Malawi's EPI was established in 1979, with support from WHO, in addition to financial contributions from donors for vaccines and cold-chain equipment, often funnelled through UNICEF. In 1998 the ICC was formed and initially focused on the Polio Eradication Initiative. (Malawi was declared polio-free in 2005.) ICC members included the Controller of Preventive Health Services and the National EPI Manager from the MoH, and numerous representatives of international agencies and bilateral donors (WHO, UNICEF, DFID, USAID, JICA (the Japanese International Cooperation Agency), NORAD, DANIDA, and KfW (the German Development Bank)) and Rotary International. Except for NORAD, these were also members of the committee that developed the GAVI application for the introduction of pentavalent vaccine.

Before GAVI was established, the situation in Malawi was similar to that in other African countries such as Uganda, with declining immunisation rates after UCI, and little interest in the introduction of new vaccines, given other health and economic priorities confronting the government (Justice 2000b). However, Malawi was among the first countries to introduce GAVI-subsidised vaccines. As part of the application process, the MoH and committee members were assisted by WHO staff and consultants. Like many other poor countries, Malawi was under pressure to meet GAVI deadlines and had to prepare its proposal without the benefit of country-specific disease burden studies, although some service-related statistics were reported to be available from Queen Elizabeth Hospital in Blantyre. The initial discussion focused on the introduction of hepatitis B, but GAVI offered Malawi only pentavalent vaccine, which included hepatitis B, DPT 1, 2, 3, and haemophilus influenzae type b vaccine (Hib). Prior to GAVI, donor organisations and the government were engaged in exploring mechanisms for government to gradually assume responsibility for payment for the six basic vaccines provided in the routine immunisation schedule. The high price of pentavalent vaccine (85% of the total vaccine budget) (Malawi Ministry of Health 2004b, p. 6) greatly increased the overall cost of the immunisation programme, thus introducing doubts related to sustainability. However, one donor representative said at the start of the process that there was little discussion about funding because the vaccines were viewed as being free (Eie 2008, p. 61). Therefore, despite the high cost of the pentavalent vaccine and the implications for long-term government funding, Malawi proceeded with the application process since GAVI was subsidising the new vaccine. The application was submitted in 2000 and pentavalent vaccine introduced in 2002.

In the early 2000s, an approach designed to integrate government health programmes, the Essential Health Package (EHP), was created, emphasising reproductive health, nutrition, and immunisation. EHP was part of the process to pool donor funding through the SWAp, which was instituted in 2004 (Malawi Ministry of Health 2004a), with the UK Department for International Development (DfID) working closely with government. The Norwegian development agency NORAD and the World Bank were also initial contributors. Because the immunisation programme was a priority both for government and donors, a form of 'earmarking' within the health SWAp was developed to ensure funding for vaccines. Around this time (2004–2005), Malawi and other countries were asked to present a plan for self-financing of pentavalent vaccine, after the initial GAVI subsidy ended. But given Malawi's economic challenges, it was not feasible for the government to pay for the new vaccine. From the government's perspective, one option was to discontinue pentavalent vaccine and continue with routine vaccines and hepatitis B, but not Hib. The global health community had a large investment in the long-term use of new vaccines and the situation was therefore resolved temporarily by an infusion of 'bridging funds' to GAVI from the BMGF (and other donors) to extend the subsidies for a period. During this time Malawi (and other governments in a similar situation) were to develop financial sustainability plans and a mechanism for co-financing (the government was to contribute US$0.20 per child vaccinated with pentavalent vaccine).

As part of the SWAp, the decision-making process in the MoH was changed. New entities were created, including the EHP Working Group (WG), and an EPI Sub-Working Group (SWG), replaced the ICC. Membership on the Working Groups also shifted, with major donors to health playing active roles on the EHP-WG, and those most directly involved with immunisation (e.g. WHO, UNICEF, USAID) represented on the EPI-SWG. For example, NORAD discontinued its representation on the EPI-SWG but continued membership on the EHP-WG. Other donors, such as DfID, are members of the EHP-WG and less directly involved with decision-making for EPI because DfID now funds GAVI, rather than funding government directly for vaccine procurement. The EPI Manager chairs the EPI-SWG on behalf of the Director of Preventive Health, to whom he reports. In addition the Malawi Medical Association, the Health Education Unit (HEU), Central Medical Stores, and representatives of district hospitals are represented on the EPI-SWG, and recently the Defence Department joined because of Malawi's participation in UN peace-keeping missions in countries with vaccine-preventable diseases. The Clinton Health Access Initiative (CHAI) is one of the few NGOs on the EPI-SWG, although there are plans to increase membership, with potential new members being the Christian Medical Association of Malawi (CHAM) and other NGOs, e.g. MSF. A major objective of the SWAp and the new WGs is to strengthen government ownership and leadership in the decision-making process, but the representation of external partners in the WGs ensures their continuing influence.

Immunisation has remained a government priority, with additional emphasis thanks to the ambition to achieve MDG4, and support available from GAVI.

Within immunisation in Malawi there has been a shift in focus from-immunisation coverage to the introduction of new vaccines, reflecting the shift at the global level noted above. Although WHO and UNICEF have retained close advisory and technical roles with government, the influence of GAVI and its public–private partners have increased. For example, while GAVI does not have an in-country presence, a key member of the GAVI Alliance (the BMGF) has recently given a three-year grant to CHAI to help facilitate the introduction of new vaccines. This provides GAVI with a substitute on-the-ground presence. Also, since 2010, Malawi has been involved in the process of introducing the current new vaccines, pnuemococcal and rotavirus vaccines. The process has not been as rushed as that of 2000–2002, when pentavalent vaccine was introduced and when GAVI, then new, was under pressure to demonstrate its effectiveness. The availability of new vaccines is viewed as a priority topic of the EPI-SWG, and more in-country data are now available about disease burden. The process of proposal development has also evolved, with EPI staff participating in regional meetings and workshops (planned and facilitated by WHO), designed to assist with the preparation of GAVI proposals. Malawi submitted proposals for both pneumococcal and rotavirus, but was told that only one new vaccine could be introduced at a time. It was decided that pneumococcal was the priority in Malawi and it was introduced in November 2011, with approval from GAVI to introduce rotavirus in 2013.

Another comparison between the introduction of new vaccines in 2002 and 2011 is related to the characteristics of the vaccines and their impact on the health system. Pentavalent vaccine fitted well with Malawi's routine immunisation schedule and its introduction was not reported to have had a major impact on the health system. In contrast, pneumococcal and rotavirus vaccines will increase the workload in an already understaffed system. They will also have a major impact on the cold chain, greatly increasing the need for cold storage space and requiring a more complex vaccine distribution system. These issues were discussed, for example a decision was made to use the GAVI funding available for health system strengthening to expand cold storage capacity at central level. It is not clear how far the perspectives of national or global participants dominated, or how the various factors were weighed in the decision-making process. Financial sustainability is a major—or even greater—concern, since both new vaccines are more expensive than pentavalent vaccine. One member of the EPI-SWG said that questions were raised about how long GAVI would continue to subsidise pentavalent vaccine (interview April 2011). Other long-term issues include the potential danger that the introduction of new vaccines could overwhelm the health system and have a negative impact on immunisation coverage. However, despite the potential negative impact on the current and future functioning of the immunisation system, in addition to concerns about long-term financial sustainability, the government of Malawi continues to accept the new vaccines as they become available. From the perspective of GAVI and the global vaccine and immunisation community, Malawi serves as a 'model' country, in contrast to criticism of its other health programmes, such as HIV/AIDS. In addition to current, and expected, future vaccine subsidies, a further incentive for Malawi to rapidly introduce new vaccines may be recognition by the global health community, manifested by the international awards it has received for its achievements related to immunisation (Nyirenda and Justice, 2012).

This brief account shows that although the government does have a role in country-level decision-making related to global health initiatives, the power of global actors is considerable. Malawi also demonstrates the risks of depending on external support, for example in 2011 when donors withheld funding for health and other sectors because of human rights issues.

India: counter expertise and activist civil society

New vaccine introduction in India contrasts in many respects with the example of Malawi. India is a middle-income country and the world's largest democracy, with 20% of the global birth cohort. When India celebrated the 60th anniversary of its constitution in 2010, however, a journalist, writing in one of the major Indian newspapers, noted the paradox that even though India's gross domestic product had increased by over 500 times since independence, the number of people below the poverty line had only fallen from 45% to 37% of the population. Even today India has 400 million people living below the poverty line (Varma 2010).

With one of the world's fastest growing economies, financial resources for paediatric immunisation are not an issue in India, and only 1.6–2% of funding comes from external sources (Sridhar and Gómez 2011). However, the GAVI Alliance has been involved in India over the past decade. India is an important country for the Alliance, reflected in a 2012 India Strategy update to the GAVI Board, where it is stressed that India has the highest birth cohort (26.6 million) of all GAVI-eligible countries, and also the largest number of unimmunised children globally (GAVI 2012). Moreover, India is considered the most important emerging country manufacturing base for vaccines, and the effects of new vaccine adoption in India on markets is therefore not to be neglected. Nevertheless, India's responses to GAVI strategies on new vaccine introduction have been subject to prolonged public debate, involving WHO, GAVI, Indian public health activists, and the Indian government. The interface between global and national perspectives in India is particularly complex.

The only new vaccines to be added to India's UIP have been against hepatitis B and Japanese encephalitis, and later against Hib disease (about which we will have more to say presently). All three new vaccines were added after the turn of the millennium. According to a government representative, decision-making on new vaccines became more structured within the MoH after 2001. In India, health and thus also immunisation is constitutionally a state responsibility. Still, central authorities set key priorities (Berman and Ahuja 2008; Sridhar and Gómez 2011). This means that decisions on new vaccines are made at the central level. The National Vaccine Policy of India describes the selection of vaccine for introduction to the UIP as a 'complex process' with 'few laid down guidelines' (MoHFW 2011, p. 17). A description of the decision-making process in the policy document does not identify a final agent of decision-making (MoHFW 2011, p. 19).

Given India's low dependency on foreign assistance to the health sector, few global organisations other than WHO, and to a more limited extent UNICEF, are involved in policy-making. A prominent exception, however, is PATH, which has had a presence in India over a long period, primarily at state level. Because of PATH's close ties to GAVI at the global level, PATH has played a role in relation to GAVI matters in India, for instance assisting in writing the GAVI application. India established a NTAGI in 2001 (John 2010). It was to bring the various stakeholders in immunisation together and formulate recommendations to the government regarding immunisation. In a research interview, a national WHO office official explained, NTAGI is 'meant to be a local expert group, for the local experts, by the local experts'.

The NTAGI is headed by the Secretary of the Ministry of Health and Family Welfare, and includes representatives from the Indian Council of Medical Research, the Indian Academy of Paediatrics, the Indian Medical Association, the government's Department of Biotechnology, and the National Drug Regulatory Authority of India. The NTAGI issues recommendations but does not make decisions. Its work is carried out by issue-specific temporary subcommittees. According to WHO representatives, global experts may be called in to assist with the scientific evidence, but the process is owned by the Indian government.

Supported by representatives of the Hib Initiative participating in discussions in the NTAGI, in December 2009 the Indian government decided it would introduce the new pentavalent Hib-containing vaccine for childhood immunisation. In January 2010, however, as a result of protests from public health activists, the decision was put on hold and it was not until the early spring of 2012 that the vaccine introduction process was set back in motion.

This situation was not widely reported internationally and it was hard for anyone to find evidence of it on GAVI or WHO websites. There had only been a news story in the *British Medical Journal*, which attributed the delay to the resistance of an 'anti-vaccine lobby' (Mudur 2010, p. 16). In India, on the other hand, the debate played out both in meetings and in Indian scientific journals. The main argument of the public health activists was that the government and public sector should establish a strong justification for immunisation through a *rational* and *evidence-based* vaccine policy, making their own policy choices independent of commercial interests. The concern was not so much about costs and financial sustainability, but rather about what is appropriate for the population, from a social and medical perspective (Madhavi et al. 2010). The public health activists argued that NTAGI overlooked evidence showing low incidence of Hib-invasive disease. Criticism dates back to the introduction of hepatitis B, when, it was claimed, proof of GAVI success was measured by the amounts of money disbursed and not the actual effects of the vaccine. Critics saw the establishment of NTAGI as a result of global pressure and placed debates about introduction of new vaccines into a larger discussion about a general policy on vaccines in India and national health security more broadly. The Indian public health activists make it clear that they are not 'antivaccine'. They endorse vaccines as a preventive medical tool. Their argument is that vaccination should not be a substitute for other basic health measures such as safe drinking water and nutrition (Madhavi et al. 2010).

The link between new vaccine introduction and domestic vaccine manufacturing is also an important dimension of the Indian debate. India has a century-old tradition of domestic manufacturing of vaccines. Traditionally, these were public sector manufacturers. Increasingly, however, private industry in India produces new vaccines for both domestic use and export. The public health activists pointed out that there has been capacity for public manufacturers to produce most of the basic six childhood vaccines, but that the gradual closure of public sector units had affected the availability and affordability of these vaccines (Madhavi et al. 2010). New vaccines, however, are produced by the private sector, and even if not included in the public immunisation programme they are available through private medical practitioners.

The relationship between government officials and public activists is not antagonistic. Since the activists are scientists and public health experts, individuals on both 'sides' are in fact professional peers, and respect the situation and dilemmas each face. The government of India is not in need of external financing, and GAVI money, as one government official stated, is more like 'oil for the machinery'. Nevertheless the Indian government has to steer a careful course. It is under pressure both to conform to global expectations of the MDGs and to navigate the domestic debate over adoption of hepatitis B, Hib and pneumococcal vaccines, which was eventually taken to the legal system. In 2009, activists filed a public interest litigation challenging the introduction of new vaccines on the basis of selective use of scientific evidence (Nair et al. 2011).

From the perspective of an NTAGI member representing the Indian government, the crux of the problem lies in the fact that India has insufficient country data as basic information for policy, and weak research capacity geared towards this task. Out of the large amounts provided by international institutions to introduce new products, if 2% of the money had been spent on generating the data, India would not have been in a situation where the issue of evidence was linked to the influence of global actors.

The recent experiences with vaccine introduction in India raise important questions of accountability. Active citizen engagement in institutions of public sector oversight is a salient feature of Indian society. The government set-up of oversight bodies and technical advisory committees can be seen as a form of horizontal accountability (Goetz and Jenkins 2011). Public confidence in these mechanisms, however, may vary. In the case of new vaccines introduced into public immunisation programmes, citizens were able to engage with the National Technical Advisory Group, also utilising the legal system as an interface with the government. In the end, citizens were able to slow down, but not stop, the elaborate decision-making machinery that makes up the world's largest democracy. The pentavalent vaccine was introduced. Indian government officials maintain that most decisions remain 'political'. Although evidence on what a 'political decision' means in reality remains opaque, this seems to imply that there is ultimately the possibility that decisions can be made or overturned at the highest level, even if contrary to recommendations and subsequent processes, if this is seen as necessary in view of other political commitments or trade-offs.

Vaccine introduction in the Netherlands

In addition to reviewing the experience of Malawi and India, it is interesting to briefly consider studies that have traced the history of vaccine introduction in the Netherlands, where several of the same issues arise: the use of evidence, the significance of economic considerations, the influence of international expertise and of public opinion (Blume and Zanders 2006; Blume and Tump 2010).

In 1971 Merck's MMR vaccine was licensed alongside the individual vaccines, and it began to be used routinely in the USA from the mid-1970s. Policy in Europe, however, was influenced by the prevailing medical opinion that mumps wasn't serious and mumps vaccination unnecessary. Despite success in controlling measles and rubella, and despite the prevailing view in the Netherlands that mumps was relatively unimportant, thereafter things began to change. First, opinion internationally was converging on the view that the purpose of vaccination against rubella should no longer be protection of individual women before they reached childbearing age, but rather reduction of virus circulation in the population as a whole. Reflecting this change of view other European countries, including the UK, were starting to vaccinate all children against rubella, and Dutch experts showed growing interest in their experiences. The increasingly international orientation led to the introduction of a new form of evidence in Dutch policy deliberation. Simulation modelling suggested that circulation of rubella virus could best be halted by vaccinating all children. In 1980 the Minister of Health requested the Health Council to advise on the desirability of immunising against mumps. When this discussion began various kinds of evidence were introduced. They included the epidemiology of the disease (its minimal fatality and limited serious consequences), but also practice in other European countries, as well as economic considerations. As discussion proceeded, and the implications of the various kinds of evidence debated, economic and international considerations became increasingly important. Rough calculations suggested that the costs of vaccinating against mumps would be more than outweighed by savings in the medical care provided to affected children. The significance of practice elsewhere was changing. By the 1980s, in suggesting that immunisation schedules in Europe might have to be standardised, government advisors were in effect internationalising the *context* in which decisions were legitimately to be made. In other words, it was no longer a question of saying 'well the evidence from France or the UK shows that the vaccine works, or that a different vaccination schedule may be better'. It was becoming a matter of saying 'other European countries are doing it like that and *therefore* we have to do the same'.

In the Netherlands pertussis vaccine had been given to almost all children since the 1950s. It was one component of the DPT (later DPTP) vaccine produced by the Institute of Public Health and included in the national immunisation programme since its beginnings in 1957. When a pertussis epidemic broke out in 1996–7 the suggestion was made that either the vaccine being used in the Netherlands was not good enough or for one reason or another it was less effective than it had been previously. An international advisory committee established by the Health Council recommended that the Netherlands should switch to the new and less reactogenic acellular vaccine, now being introduced in many developed countries. It was argued that the Netherlands seemed at that time the only country with such an epidemic, whilst many countries had already changed over to acellular vaccine. In 2000, the apparently declining efficacy of the existing vaccine was once more an issue, and in 2004 the Health Council again recommended that the Netherlands switch completely to the acellular vaccine. Despite the fact that local vaccinologists were not convinced that acellular pertussis vaccine was the long-term answer for the Netherlands, experience abroad was taken as proving its superiority. Finally, in 2005, the Minister of Health announced that acellular vaccine would be introduced.

If we look across these vaccine introductions we see a major shift. In the 1960s, despite international preference for the live OPV, the Netherlands' own experience in controlling polio, and avoiding unnecessary changes to the immunisation schedule, were over-riding considerations. By the 1980s, when the Health Council (at the request of the Minister of Health) was debating a possible change to the rubella immunisation strategy, and the desirability of starting mumps vaccination, new arguments were introduced. For one thing, economic considerations were starting to weigh more heavily. For another, growing importance was being attached to epidemiological studies done in other countries, published in the international literature and forming the basis for professional consensus internationally. Thus, despite studies carried out in the Netherlands in the early 1980s suggesting little difference in efficacy between the two rubella vaccines, international opinion carried the day. Debate around the two pertussis vaccines, some years later, shows much the same, although here public opinion also played an important role in influencing the political decision.

Set against our studies of Malawi and India, the Netherlands case suggests that despite the differences in concerns, there are also similarities in the influences coming to bear. We see a growing emphasis on evidence-informed decision-making, and that evidence is becoming increasingly similar internationally.

Conclusions

The availability of new children's vaccines coupled with an increase in funding for the poorest countries through the GAVI Alliance have been key to bringing about a shift from a focus on immunisation coverage to a focus on new vaccine introduction. Data on levels of funding show that this has become the global priority. The rates at which GAVI-eligible countries introduce new vaccines suggest that national level priorities have come to reflect global ones. But while policy decisions made at the global level may be grounded in collective wisdom, the challenge lies in ensuring their implementation at the national level. The terminology in global health publications on vaccine introduction is revealing, with concepts like 'political will', 'ensuring political buy in', 'accelerating introduction', 'shaping the market', and 'antivaccine lobby'. Expressions such as these affirm the expectations that national governments respond positively to global objectives. There is indeed, potentially, a virtuous cycle of reaching more children with immunisation, increasing production volumes, spurring competition, and eventually bringing prices down, enabling more countries access.

In this chapter we have been concerned with national responses to the global prioritisation of new vaccine introduction. We began with a number of questions to better understand how processes of vaccine introduction work at the country level. We have seen how global bodies, GAVI in particular, do not simply say 'support for the introduction of this or that new vaccine is available', and then sit back and wait for countries to respond. They try to create 'political will', just as Jim Grant had once said they should. When the pentavalent vaccine, containing Hib antigen, became available, country responses were viewed as too slow. GAVI, as we saw, then established the Hib Initiative to muster evidence and mobilise support at the country level. The result was that the proportion of GAVI-eligible countries adopting the new vaccine rose rapidly. At the same time, countries have been assisted in establishing NTAGIs and where specific national evidence is lacking they have been advised to show greater willingness to accept regional data instead (Scott Jordon et al. 2012).

The comparison of decision-making in Malawi and in India is revealing. Although both countries did introduce the pentavalent vaccine, the processes were quite different. In Malawi global actors, particularly major donor countries, are deeply involved in decision-making at the national level. The availability of evidence seems to have played little part. Kaul has argued, as we saw earlier, that for many low-income countries, rejecting international interference is not an option, since it carries the risk of losing the support on which they rely (Kaul 2006). They have to be responsive to global policies. This seems to be the case in Malawi, where 60% of healthcare expenditure comes from external sources. As long as donors are forthcoming, the implicit perception seems to be that vaccines are affordable. In reality, the government is dependent on external funding and on vaccine prices, neither of which it controls. In Malawi, there is limited citizen engagement in decision-making, very limited accountability to citizens, and an absence of domestic vaccine supplies. And Malawi adopts new vaccines very rapidly: much more rapidly than many richer countries, including India, our other case study.

India differs in a number of crucial respects. One is its financial independence. Another is the existence of a large domestic industry producing vaccines. Both these factors make India far less dependent on global actors. No less important is the country's vibrant civil society and long tradition of political activism, which led to the disputes around the 1994 Surat plague outbreak and the PATH HPV study discussed in Chapter 2. Indian public health activists demanded that if Hib vaccine were to be introduced in India, this should be done on the basis of national medical evidence showing that the vaccine was needed, and not in response to global pressure. Nor was vaccination to be used as a substitute for other much-needed public health measures.

Children benefit from increased immunisation coverage and, potentially, from the new vaccines. So does the pharmaceutical industry through increasing vaccine sales, global health initiatives through having their objectives met, and national governments through fulfilling the expectations of both the international and national communities. Governments have a specific role in relation to vaccines as negotiating terms of engagement with the population. They have discretionary power in relation to global immunisation initiatives, since their efforts determine success or failure, but the degree of that discretionary power differs from country to country. It depends on the country's dependence on donor resources for health, and it depends on the functioning of civil society and the availability of (counter) expertise in the community. A study of the global–national interface reveals a bias in the global community in favour of immunisation as a cost-effective tool with measurable results. Debate arises when governments or citizens see that preventing the same diseases may be just as feasible with other tools that require a different modus operandi by national governments than responding to global policies.

In light of the observations of India and Malawi, juxtaposed with findings from other studies, we return to the question: Is there a national perspective on new vaccine introduction? From the global discourse, one easily identifies a distinct set of objectives, even one vision that drives efforts on immunisation, namely equal global access to life-saving vaccines. At the national level, we conclude simply that there are multiple perspectives, as many as there are nation states. The conclusion may appear obvious, but it begs the follow-up question of whether global initiatives are fully capable of grasping this diversity. There is an emerging emphasis on the importance of evidence-based decision-making, not only in high-income countries but also in GAVI-eligible countries. If taken seriously—and this is the argument made by the Indian public health activists—this would strengthen country ownership. Embracing country ownership, however, assumes that states will act in the interest of their citizens. Therefore the crucial question is: What counts as evidence and how do governments and politicians act on it? Is it reasonable to rely on regional evidence when national evidence is lacking? Who is to supply the evidence, given the important role of international experts in many national decision-making processes? How should one measure the success of new vaccine introduction, taking into account the impact of new technology on existing immunisation systems, cold chains and health systems more generally, matters of which little is known and of which few studies have been carried out?

We conclude that national processes of new vaccine introduction differ, and often in what appears to be a paradoxical way; that in a country with strong civil society participation, a relatively advanced economy, a relatively good evidence base and expertise, and a local vaccine industry, resistance to global recommendations to introduce a new vaccine is more likely to emerge than in one that does not.

Chapter 5

Rights and obligations in national health governance

Sidsel Roalkvam and Jagrati Jani

Introduction

States gain legitimacy through performance—the support, protection, and public services they provide to their people. When President Mutharika of Malawi, a former World Bank economist, was first elected in 2004 he represented himself and his office to his constituency by benevolent health messages. All over the country there were huge billboards advertising the face of the new President and his message to the people: 'let's join hands against AIDS', 'Drive safely', and 'Vaccinate your child'. President Mutharika launched Malawi's first National AIDS Policy. Foreign donors, responsible for a large share of the state budget, regarded this as a very timely message in a country where little attention was paid to the escalating AIDS crisis. This policy set the goal of improving the provision of prevention, treatment, care, and support services, and called for a multisectoral response to the epidemic.

In this chapter our focus is on state practices concerning immunisation, and more generally people's health. We are concerned with how the state negotiates its priorities to provide health interventions, how material, resources, and personnel are organised and distributed to regional and community level, in organisational terms but also—more concretely—through the infrastructure of the cold chain. Health services are, as we shall see, crucial for the political legitimacy of the state. But contemporary scholars see the state as in a profound transformative crisis (Shore 2001; Troulliot 2001), losing its autonomy not only to an ever-expanding market, but also to a number of initiatives by external, global actors. Marchall and Cavalli (2009) see the dramatic change in the landscape of public health brought about by the explosion of new global health initiatives as severely limiting a state's capacity to govern and develop its own national health priorities and health systems. They criticise the health MDGs, for example, as short-term initiatives directed at specific diseases with an easily demonstrated outcome that can be achieved within a short timeframe. In these critics' view, the MDGs are designed to fulfil the requirements of donors concerned with global objectives and applying instruments targeted to reach a population identified as 'the global poor'. Aid is misaligned with the actual needs of countries, it is argued; chronic long-term health problems and their social and economic determinants are least likely to be addressed by the current health programmes. As discussed in Chapter 4, with reference to Kaul (2006), the national governance space has since the 1990s been heavily impacted by the proliferation of external policy expectations, raising new visions and creating new demands. In Chapter 4 we saw how national policy-makers need to blend demands from external and domestic sources. In this chapter we bring this discussion one step further and explore how these policy blends affect the priorities and performances within national health systems, focusing as before on MDG4.

A policy intervention such as immunisation involves a myriad of challenges. Although the main aim is benevolent—protecting the people against threats to their health—this is also where the formal power of the state is brought to bear (Brown 2010, p. 161). In the practice of public health there is an inherent contrast between an image of people as 'citizens' (rights bearers making legitimate demands) on the one hand and as 'the population' (targets of state projects) on the other. Inherent to the concept of population is to see people as identifiable, classifiable, and describable as members of particular segments and groups. Chatterjee (2004) rightfully suggests that:

> Unlike the concept of citizens which carries the ethical connotation of participation in the sovereignty of the state, the concept of population makes available to governmental functionaries a set of rationally manipulable instruments for reaching larger sections of the inhabitants of a country as they target their 'policies'. (Chatterjee 2004, p. 8)

The rhetoric of prevailing global and national policy statements in health portrays the state's relationship to its citizens in a humanitarian light. Yet people often give very little priority to preventive health measures such as immunisation. Preference is given to health interventions that help people recover, not to those that keep them from falling ill in the first place. Governments responsive to their citizenry are thus inclined to give first priority to cure and care. Population-based health interventions such as immunisation often lead to disputes about the legitimate role of the state in relation to the citizen and the relative weight of social and individual responsibility. Since the benefits of vaccination are much greater if everyone is vaccinated, many argue that it is the responsibility of the citizen to vaccinate his or her child. On the other hand, others criticise coercion of any kind and argue that to accept a vaccine or not should be a matter of individual choice. Essentially this boils down to personal liberty vs the good of the society. This deeply ethical and political question tends to be recast as a scientific, technical problem set within a system of rational practices of government referred to by Chatterjee—beyond the realm of politics, as it were. The technologies that are applied gain legitimacy from various types of expert knowledge, and the issue of accountability is transformed into simple, transparent, and objectively measurable indicators of numbers of children vaccinated: maximising this number becomes the right thing to do.

The situation is complicated, however, by several factors. One is that accountability to a global audience may be based on a very different logic when a disease becomes a threat beyond national borders. Secondly, an epidemic may change people's attitudes; a sudden outbreak of disease may generate an urgent demand for immunisation that was not previously there, and cause people to hold the state accountable if it fails to deliver. It is particularly revealing to study what happens in such situations which serve as 'natural experiments capable of illuminating fundamental patterns of social value and institutional practice', as historian of medicine Charles Rosenberg has noted (Rosenberg 1992, p. 279). 'For the social scientist, epidemics constitute an extraordinarily useful sampling device', 'Just as a playwright chooses a theme and manages plot development', he goes on, 'so a particular society constructs its characteristic response to an epidemic.' Before doing this, however, we will first describe in some detail the technology of vaccine supply; how the system is supposed to work, this 'clean vertical intervention', as it was described by one of our interviewees, an MoH official in India.

Distributing vaccines: the cold chain

The health benefits of immunisation are to a large degree dependent on achieving relatively high coverage among cohort after cohort of children. The vaccine infrastructure is first and foremost a governmental responsibility. With new vaccine introductions countries are facing the challenge of maintaining cost-effective, high-quality supply chains as more temperature-sensitive products are introduced. National immunisation programmes can only function when a specific set of inputs—vaccines—are available on a reliable basis. The routes the vaccines travel from the manufacturer to the child to be vaccinated depend crucially on what is known as the 'cold chain', and a vast network of the chains is to be found in any country with an EPI programme. In this section we are going to journey along such a route in order to properly understand the complexities of cold-chain logistics and management. The cold chain is a concrete chain of immunisation depots, buildings and refrigerators, freezers and coolers that branches out from the national to the regional and the local level. Yet vaccine programmes have long struggled with what seems to be a straightforward problem: keeping the vaccines cold. Nearly all vaccines are thermally unstable: 97% of vaccines need to be stored between 2 and 8°C in order to maintain their efficacy (Galazka et al. 2006). The cold chain is the spine of the immunisation system, but also one of its most vulnerable parts. Cold-chain 'breaks' can lead to ineffective vaccines being administered. When vaccine failure is detected, either by serological studies of vaccinated populations or by the occurrence of cases in a supposedly vaccinated population, the cause is most likely to be a breakdown in the cold chain, and this most often happens near the end of the chain. Some important varieties of vaccine and sera are inactivated even at room temperature in temperate zones, and in hot tropical regions they are not only inactivated, but some may even become toxic (see Figure 5.1).

The fragile nature of vaccines thus means that they need to be kept at the correct temperature as they are passed along the supply chain. India's UIP is one of the largest vaccine programmes in the world in terms of quantities of vaccines used, the number of beneficiaries, the number of immunisation sessions organised, and the geographical spread and diversity of areas covered; the logistic challenges are tremendous just by virtue of its size. The UIP in India targets 27 million infants and 30.2 million pregnant women. Immunisation services are provided through a vast healthcare infrastructure numbering 618 district hospitals, 4045 community health centres, 22,395 primary health centres (PHCs), and 144,988 subcentres (UNICEF 2008). Although not entirely part of it, the cold chain follows structure of the health system. In India vaccines are transported through a four-tier vaccine store network: from the manufacturer to governmental medical store depots, further on to divisional vaccine stores, then on to district, and finally to community health centres (CHC) and PHCs. The last-named are fixed immunisation points or door-to-door immunisation. At the periphery of the cold chain vaccines are distributed to small clinics in insulated polystyrene boxes packed in dry ice. During vaccination sessions the stored vaccines must be kept at a suitable low temperature at all times, and only enough for use on people actually awaiting vaccination should be removed from refrigeration at one time (see Figure 5.2).

A fully immunised child in India is protected against six vaccine-preventable diseases (VPD), tuberculosis, diphtheria, tetanus, pertussis, polio, and measles, and will have received a BCG vaccine, three doses of OPV, three doses of DPT, and one dose of measles in the eligible population (12–23 months of age) and at the correct time. The first DPT should be given before 6 weeks and measles antigen at less than 9 months. The percentages of children who have received the third dose of DPT is thus frequently used as a proxy for full immunisation in reporting coverage. The vaccination schedule (the series of vaccinations,

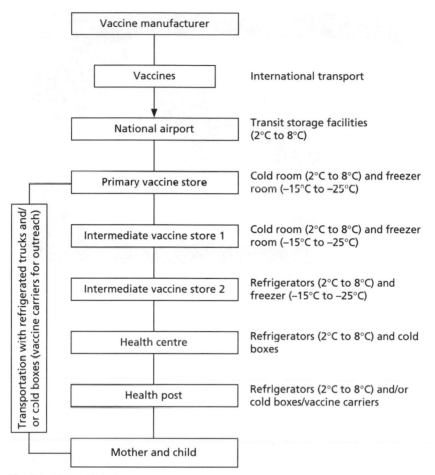

Fig. 5.1 The cold chain.

Adapted by Oxford University Press with permission, from Module 3: *The Cold Chain in Immunization in Practice: A Practical Resource Guide for Health Workers*, 2004 Update, Figure 3A, available from http://www.who.int/vaccines-documents/iip/PDF/Module3.pdf (accessed 30 October 2012).

including the timing of all doses, recommended or compulsory) is the foundation for vaccine supply and cold-chain logistics. It follows from this that introduction of new vaccines has a tremendous effect on cold-chain logistics: it affects the size of depots and of stores, the size and number of freezers needed, and may require alterations in the vaccine schedule that demand retraining of health workers and re-education of mothers. The most recent cold-chain assessments in both India and Malawi have been to prepare for new vaccine introduction. GAVI funds for health system strengthening have been used in both India and Malawi to improve cold-chain facilities. New combination vaccines (vaccines

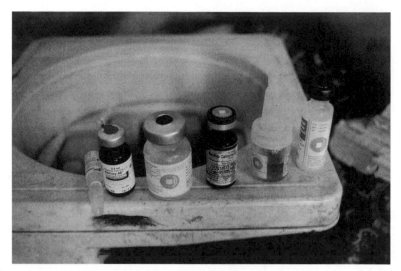

Fig. 5.2 The cold box used for distributing vaccines to health posts.
Photo: Courtesy of Dagrun Kyte Gjøstein.

consisting of two or more different vaccines that have been combined into a single shot) can have a positive effect on cold-chain constraints.

When the EPI was launched in India in 1978 it was, as a Ministry of Health and Family Welfare (MoHFW) official put it, a 'clean vertical intervention'. It gained impetus under the UIP and was carried out in a phased manner to cover all districts in the country by 1989–90 (MoHFW 2006, p. 58) Under the UIP, vaccines for six vaccine preventable diseases are available free of charge for all. More than 90 million pregnant women and 83 million infants were to be immunised over a 5-year period under the UIP. The programme was given the status of a National Technology Mission in 1986 (Government of India 1988) to provide a sense of urgency and commitment to achieve the goals within the specified period. The expansion of the UIP, however, was not followed by strengthening cold-chain logistics management and equipment.

During our period of research there was one cold-chain issue that puzzled us. Although the Indian government procured vaccines estimated on the basis of 100% coverage, free of charge to all children in all individual states, official coverage could be as low as 35% in some districts (Sharma 2007). Although full immunisation increased to 51.8% of children aged 12–23 months in Orissa, for example, 58% remain unanswered for (Government of India 2006). In order to pursue this puzzle we decided to travel along the cold chain from the governmental medical store to the periphery of the cold chain, to the vaccinator with her cooler box, interviewing cold-chain managers and staff, referred to as 'the cold-chain guys', on the way. The Government of India Multi Year Strategic plan 2005–2010, on UIP specifically, directed our attention as to where to look. This report concluded that vaccine cold-chain logistics was an acute problem. The plan noted that coverage was not uniform. There was poor implementation of the programme, poor monitoring, high drop-out rates, over-reporting, staff vacancies, and poor maintenance of equipment. There were faults along the entire chain. Wastage was high and not monitored at all. In 2008 the Government of India followed up and conducted a cold-chain assessment in collaboration with WHO and UNICEF. The assessment took stock of the situation and assessed the capacity of the current cold chain to accommodate the introduction of additional or new vaccines. It painted a rather bleak picture. The cold chain suffered from an acute shortage of specialised staff who could manage cold-chain logistics at all levels of the system. The current tedious practice of recording, reporting, and procurement of cold-chain equipment, spare parts, vaccines, and logistics prevents appropriate supply chain management and timely forecasting, with serious stock out situations as a result (UNICEF and National Rural Health Mission 2008). When we journeyed the cold chain in 2010, new buildings with new freezers with UNICEF labels on them had been installed in central vaccine stores at national and state level but from there to the periphery the situation remained as before. At all levels—apart from the national—the main problem was identified as the supply of vaccines. As will be discussed in Chapter 6, a regular complaint amongst health workers was failure to supply a sufficient quantity of vaccines to the point of delivery and at the right time. The reason for this could be traced back all the way up the chain to the procedures for procurement. The national level of UIP assumed 100% coverage in passing vaccines down into the system, but without taking any account of cold-chain constraints within the individual states. Under the Indian Constitution, health is largely the responsibility of the states, but the national government finances national public health programmes that have high social returns or are characterised as public goods, and UIP is one of these. However, and crucially, although the national government provides the vaccines, the funds for maintaining the cold-chain infrastructure remain the responsibility of the individual state. Hence the cold chain has to compete with other health priorities within the tight budgets of the individual state.

Maintaining the cold chain is thus a complex matter. Cold-chain planning involves immunisation operations such as service delivery, the logistics of vaccines and infrastructure, purchase of refrigerators and other material, quality control of vaccines, and communication in support of the programme. In more detail this involves an overview of the space and size of the buildings needed as well as the transport necessary for the total vaccine supply for every child each month. It is a continuing struggle to secure enough space and refrigerators needed for stocks. In theory the UIP managers are supposed to organise refresher courses on cold-chain maintenance, and distribution and administration of the vaccines. In practice there is an acute shortage of properly trained staff. In order to succeed in timely distribution of vaccines the cold chain also involves trucks, drivers, and coolers. Vaccine availability thus was also vulnerable to shortages of trained staff, absence of staff, shortages of drivers, trucks and coolers, bad roads, and rainy seasons. Operating and providing an immunisation system demands professional staff at all levels of the chain with solid knowledge regarding the preservation of vaccine quality, the monitoring range of temperatures for each type of vaccines, calculation of vaccine coverage rates, the correct immunisation schedule, vaccine safety issues, and more technical aspects of good maintenance and repair of refrigerators and freezers.

India faces a tremendous challenge in reaching all her children; coverage surveys show an average achievement of only 62.4% (MoHFW Family Welfare Statistics in India 2006). Although the serious situation of a weak, understaffed cold chain is well known to health planners and policy-makers, the pressure on community health workers to achieve the targets of coverage continues. Under the National Rural Health Mission (NRHM), launched in 2004, the policy chosen was not to first secure the cold-chain infrastructure in order to improve coverage but to invest in a new cadre of community health workers (Accredited Social Health Activists, ASHAs) whose main responsibility is to mobilise community members to vaccinate their children. Each ASHA is paid 100 rupees (the equivalent to US$I.8) for every full vaccination schedule he or she is able to perform. That the supply of vaccines is in fact unreliable has become a problem left to the community health workers and mothers to solve. At every interface of the cold chain, blame was shifted downward. The national government blamed the individual state, the individual state blamed the health workers, and the health workers blamed the mothers for not attending immunisation days, although more often than not no vaccines were available.

Any cold chain in the developing world gives rise to similar logistical problems, and cold-chain management is crucial and complex. Since high rates of immunity can only be attained with properly preserved vaccines, a substantial part of the vaccine literature dealing with the developing world is concerned with cold-chain management, logistics, and failures. There are significant economic consequences if the cold chain is broken, for example a refrigerator full of the more expensive combination vaccines can contain many thousands of dollars' worth of vaccines. Even more importantly, vaccines damaged by exposure to temperatures that are too high or too low affect the protection of the children vaccinated. Confidence in immunisation can be greatly harmed when children vaccinated with an ineffective vaccine subsequently get the disease. As we shall see below, cold-chain breaks can affect an entire population if they lead to disease outbreaks. It remains a puzzle that whilst vaccination coverage is so high a priority, cold-chain maintenance and logistics—so crucial to success— still receive so little attention.

Crises and epidemics

Health has become an index not only of the economic progress of nations but also of the legitimacy of governments. It has become important for governments in both the developed and developing world to show that they care for their citizens, and the adequacy of health services show that they do so. Their efforts come under particular scrutiny during diseases outbreaks. As noted in the introduction to this chapter, epidemics are instructive for social scientists because they offer special insights into the social values and institutional practices of a society. Whereas governments can deal with normal and anticipated 'crises' that become routinised over a prolonged period of time, sudden outbreaks are different. The routinisation of crisis is exemplified by the occurrence of cholera epidemics in India. Here cholera has been articulated as chronic crisis by the state and a 'normal crisis' by local communities (Das and Dasgupta 2000; Ghosh and Coutinho 2000). By contrast, faced with a rapid outbreak of measles, for example, the need for the state to control the situation becomes urgent and more fraught with risk to public order, to collective benefit, and to state legitimacy.

The medical anthropologist Andrew Lakoff (2010) argues that new emerging disease threats, combined with a weakening public health system, have marked a troubling reversal in the history of public health. At the moment when it seemed that vaccines had succeeded in taking control of infectious disease we are witnessing a return of the 'microbe': diseases of the underdeveloped world. The AIDS crisis, the influenza pandemics, and seemingly new diseases such as SARS or ebola are all examples of this. Countries need to control outbreaks not only to protect their own citizens but also the citizens of the world. In this context it is instructive to observe the responses when Dr Margaret Chan, Director-General of WHO, announced the emergence of a novel influenza A (H1N1) in June 2009. She did so in a global environment in which it was asserted that effective vaccines were becoming available, and a newly developed set of global health regulations should help countries respond. The virus was contagious, spreading easily from one person to another and from one country to another. Considering the 30,000 confirmed cases reported in 74 countries, and that these were, with few exceptions, countries with good surveillance and testing procedures in place, WHO proclaimed that 'the world was at the start of the 2009 influenza pandemic' (WHO 2009e) and called urgently for planned mitigation efforts. Dr Chan's announcement led to different responses in different countries: responses that reflect the varying social and political contexts within which such an announcement is translated into action. A few examples illustrate this.

In oil-rich Norway the health authorities responded to Dr Chan's announcement by proclaiming that they would start a mass vaccination programme costing US$650 million. The Norwegian Minister of Health announced that 10,000 Norwegians could possibly die and urged citizens to respond positively to the vaccination campaign. He also approved 400 respirators to be bought from the state health budget to meet the need for respiratory support for infected Norwegians. Commentators in local Norwegian media asked him to calm down. They argued that mild winter flu was something all Norwegians were prepared for. Nor were they convinced by the Minister of Health's argument that it was thanks to Norway's good global connections that so swift a response was possible. In fact the public were sceptical, seeing exactly these connections as the reason why the nation felt the need to spend so much money on something for which there would probably be no need. Bloggers questioned if it was not all a scam put into motion by the 'vaccine mafia'. In the early days of the H1N1 outbreak only one in five Norwegians was willing to be vaccinated. The low response rate worried state health officials, who urged people to protect not only themselves but others as well. One healthcare official went so far as to appeal to Norwegians' patriotic duty, thus highlighting the citizens' responsibility in pandemic control. News commentators were sceptical, however, and looked upon the Norwegian Minister of Health as someone most eager to please his friends in WHO and GAVI. It was also suggested that he was scared of being accused of not doing enough to prevent illness, as an election was coming up. He was continuously reminded that malaria is still the world's largest health problem, killing 125 people every hour in Africa, Asia, and South America, and that AIDS killed 150,000 last week hence he was confusing, as it were, his priorities. But when an image of a seriously ill 15-year-old boy in a respirator appeared on the front page of Norwegian newspapers public opinion rapidly changed. Overnight attitudes shifted from indifference to panic. Even the well-functioning Norwegian health system felt the pressure of increased demand and turned out to be as vulnerable as any other to the limitations of global vaccine supply. As it turned out, Western governments had to admit that they had been widely optimistic in estimating vaccine availability. The reliance on old production processes led to a severe shortage of the H1N1 vaccine. It also became clear that political influence and power, not vulnerability or need, determined the allocation of the limited supply.

In India, the health ministry also responded, leaving no stone unturned in response to Dr Chan's call. Cabinet Secretary KM Chandrasekhar of the Indian government also chose a highly visible reaction when he promptly decided to install thermal scanners at Delhi's Indira Gandhi international airport to screen out suspected influenza H1N1 cases coming in from affected countries. The scanner was designed to detect a person having an above-normal body temperature, thus checking the import of the infection into the country. The Delhi administration followed up by forming nine rapid-response groups and assigning 11 state hospitals as treatment centres to deal with new H1N1 influenza cases. Mr J P Singh, Principal Secretary (Health) in the Delhi Government, said that infected persons were to be admitted to the Airport Health Organization hospital at the airport. 'We can't leave infected people at their homes. We have invoked the Epidemic Diseases Act, 1897, under which no H1N1 infected person can stay at home. We can't leave infected people at their homes,' he announced (Cittangia 2010). Thus the government invoked the Epidemic Diseases Act, 1897, under which extraordinary measures could be taken in order to protect the population. India had at this point reported 16 cases of the flu. Researchers from the Defence Research and Development Organization (DRDO) quickly developed a blood test kit that could detect H1N1 virus within an hour.

The Cabinet Secretary of India was reacting to a history of national epidemic outbreaks and heavy criticism of the government's ability to respond to crisis. In Chapter 2 we discussed briefly the 1994 outbreak of plague in India. The notion of crisis was central to structuring state responses. A study done by Addlakha (2001) analyses why Indian governments have tended to exercise caution in designating disease outbreak as epidemics. In the 1996 outbreak of dengue fever in Delhi the government was heavily criticised for not enforcing the Diseases Act, a factor believed to explain the slow and poorly coordinated response. In the public debates concerned with the 1996 outbreak of dengue fever and the court's ruling on the government's neglect, several reasons were given to explain the actions of the authorities. First, keeping the 1994 plague in mind, the government was afraid of creating panic. Second, such a move would adversely affect tourism and trade. Third, the government might wish to avoid a focus on loopholes in state health policies, particularly in the case of dengue fever and the issue of sanitation. Fourth and last, all the above needed to be avoided in order to win the next election! So in the case of the dengue fever outbreak, although more than 3300 cases were reported, the health minister tried to have it both ways, stating 'I would not call it an epidemic although the efforts we are making are of epidemic proportions' (*The Hindustan Times* 16 October 1996, quoted in Addlakha 2001).

In Egypt the government responded to Dr Chan's announcement by deciding to kill the pigs of the garbage collectors in Cairo. This is a minority Christian group in a majority Muslim society, which makes a livelihood with its pigs by collecting Cairo's trash and transforming it into a commodity. International agencies quickly criticised the authorities, saying that pigs were not spreading the illness, but Egypt did not stop the huge pig cull. Egypt, which had no swine flu cases, was the only country in the world to order a mass pig slaughter in response to the disease. The move mirrored Egypt's response to bird flu, in which the government killed 25 million birds within weeks in 2006. But the Egyptian government was also acting in a political landscape where it was important that the government appeared strong and proactive in the swine flu scare, having taken heavy criticism at home for poor planning and corruption during past crises. When ridiculed in local newspapers for taking measures that even WHO did not approve, the government proclaimed that it was no longer acting just to prevent swine flu, but that it was carrying out part of a plan to clean up and finally get the garbage collectors to live in sanitary conditions (apparently ignoring the function that the pigs served as garbage collectors in a city with poor public services).

It is clear from the above examples that a country's decision to declare an epidemic is not based on merely technical grounds and has profound administrative and political implications. Vaccine availability is a political issue. It is subject to authority, power, and control often beyond the control of national governments. But vaccine supply and availability within countries can in some instances also be an issue, critically evaluated by specific groups in terms of fairness, equity, and justice. Shortage of vaccines in such circumstances could be interpreted as unfair health service distribution (Vaughan and Tinker 2009). When the Norwegians panicked and vaccine shortage was a fact under the N1H1 outbreak it became hugely controversial that the health authorities shipped vaccines to the north of the country when the south was seen as more vulnerable. Anger and frustration loomed amongst people lining up for vaccines, unsure if there would be any left when their turn came. It seemed that the Norwegian authorities were not on top of the situation. Thus, even in a situation where trust in the authorities is high, it can be eroded during a disease outbreak. Trust in the authorities is central to how the public hear, interpret, and respond to public health messages. As discussed in Chapter 2, in Nigeria the eradication of polio has been understood as a threat to Muslim minorities rather than a benevolent protective measure. Likewise, the killing of pigs in Cairo was immediately interpreted as a measure to control and even perhaps demean a religious minority. Epidemic messages speak directly into a specific socioeconomic and cultural context within which these messages are understood. For all governments, not only those of the developing world, an emergency such as an epidemic outbreak provides a challenge to state legitimacy. The responsibility of the state for the outbreak of disease in the body-politic is indeed articulated in times of such crisis. Governments are seen as responsible for protecting the body-politic. In addition, both strengths and weaknesses of governance are exposed during an epidemic outbreak. Maintaining political stability during a disease outbreak is a balancing act. In order to gain control over the situation, to get citizens to act in accordance with an epidemic protocol, the authorities need both to build trust and to dispel rumours. And the public demands that the government is taking control over the epidemic. Learning from the 2009 H1N1 outbreak, the USA, under the Department of Homeland Security and the Department of Health and Human Services, in January 2010 launched a National Health Security Strategy: the first comprehensive strategy focusing on protecting people's health during large-scale emergencies.

The global policy focus on disease surveillance and outbreak control has made infectious disease a security issue, motivated by the desire to protect workforce, consumers, trading interests, and national borders. Because they are geographically concentrated far from developed countries and hence not perceived as important threats, some diseases receive little attention. Endemic cholera in India, for example, does not impinge much on the rest of the world. Homeland defence is concerned with disease threats across borders rather than with the illnesses producing the most fatalities. But in the era of global health, a government's response to a pandemic is meant not only to protect its own citizens but also to protect the citizens of the world. Disease surveillance protects citizens but it also protects the status of states among states. Which country would wish to be labelled as the origin of a world threat? When India—a country that in 2009 had more polio cases than any other country in the world—was taken off the WHO polio list, the *Times of India* captured this sense of national unease when it proclaimed on its front page 'India's name has been struck off the shame list that the country hope will never include it in the future' (*Times of India*, 26 February 2012).

Immunisation is thus a national preventive state practice that moves beyond the nation state. Disease control has become protection also against global threats that pay no heed to national borders. India's containment of polio also resulted in an increased surveillance against polio along the line of control bordering Pakistan, which has had a major increase in polio cases. In the case of H1N1, a modest outbreak as it turned out, Indian colleagues were amazed by the energy and accuracy with which public health officers conducted their preventive tasks at the country's major airports—despite being baffled about the options available to them if any person entered the country with an 'above normal temperature'. The fact that at this point India had reported 16 cases of the flu contrasted cruelly with the fact that the country at that time had the world's greatest burden of maternal, newborn, and child deaths. She also had the greatest number of malnourished children. There are 52 million stunted children in India, and the range and burden of infectious disease is enormous (Balarajan et al. 2011; Horton and Das 2011; Rao et al. 2011; Sengupta and Prasad 2011). Health priorities have become part of a country's foreign policy portfolio, with major implications for those determining them in the individual nation states.

We have seen in the above paragraphs the need for governments to be visible and proactive in a situation of a pandemic outbreak as if their political legitimacy is dependent on it. We shall now look more closely at a specific case—a measles outbreak in one of the world's most aid-dependent countries. In what follows we will see how Malawian authorities tried to secure some kind of visibility as a proactive government during the crisis.

A measles outbreak

In terms of gross national product Malawi is the second poorest country in the world, but it has nevertheless become known for its impressive immunisation coverage. UNICEF ranks Malawi first, together with Gambia and Mauritius, in subSaharan countries for their 90% coverage of the DPT 3 vaccine (UNICEF 2012). As in most other subSaharan African countries, Malawi includes EPI in its chosen essential health package (EHP), which is seen as the health sector's contribution to the MDG of poverty reduction. Malawi has also succeeded in boosting immunisation coverage against measles from only 50% in 1980 to almost 90% in 1999 (World Health Organization 2000). As a result, the number of reported cases and deaths fell dramatically. During 1999, only two laboratory-confirmed cases were reported, and, for the first time ever, no measles deaths. However, in 2010 the Malawian government launched an extensive measles immunisation drive in response to the worst epidemic that had been witnessed in the country in almost 10 years. No fewer than 77,000 measles cases and 195 deaths were recorded in the period between January and March 2010 (Karat 2010). The measles outbreak was looked on as a crisis of the vertical EPI programme. It revealed invisible facets of the EPI and raised questions as to whether the high vaccine coverage figures that had been reported over the years were reliable. In 2009 and 2010, 642 and 118,712 cases of measles were reported (World Health Organization 2012).

The Malawian government responded by using its power to initiate a US$4.2 million crusade. Health Ministry spokesperson Storn Kabuluzi said that six million children, aged up to 15 years, were targeted by the mass immunisation campaign launched by the government. Children ran the highest risk of dying in the outbreak since in the previous decade they had not received a second dose of measles vaccine because of shortages, according to Kabuluzi.

Malawi's MoH worked in partnership with Médecins Sans Frontières (MSF) in providing medical support to hospitals and health centres located in both rural and urban areas in caring for measles patients. MSF support ranged from reinforcing and training medical staff to donations of medicines and equipment. In order to prevent further worsening of the epidemic, MSF and the MoH launched several mass vaccination campaigns.

Malawi's health system is deficient under normal conditions and moreover heavily dependent on aid. WHO estimates that about 60% of total health expenditure comes from external sources (World Health Organization 2009e). Three agencies provide health services in Malawi: the MoH, which provides 60%, followed by the Christian Health Association of Malawi (CHAM) at 37%, while private institutions provide the remaining 3%. The MoH in Malawi has two departments that deal with the healthcare system: the Planning and Preventive Departments. Within the healthcare system there are different programmes, such as HIV and AIDS, EPI, Safe Motherhood, Maternal and Child Health, malaria, and others. Four levels constitute the health delivery system: central hospitals, district hospitals, health centres, and community-based outreach care.

Global health objectives were to be realised within the SWAp, a system designed by donors and the MoH to improve priority setting and health system performance, and hence the ability to meet MDG targets. The SWAp is an arrangement whereby donor funding from different agencies is pooled in support of a shared sector-wide policy and strategy for implementation. Ideally this should be done under governmental leadership in a sustained partnership with the multiple donors. The aim of the SWAp is to deliver an EHP, a clearly defined and costed package of key interventions that will serve as the basis for pooled funding to the health sector (Malawi Ministry of Health 2004a; UNICEF 2011; Nyirenda and Flikke 2012). This EHP should address the major causes of morbidity and mortality in the country: vaccine preventable disease, malaria, maternal and child health, tuberculosis, acute respiratory infections, and HIV and AIDS. The EPI, launched in Malawi in 1979, is one of the programmes that now functions under the SWAp, although because it has high priority it has earmarked funds within the SWAp. All agencies/institutions provide EPI services at all levels. As of 2005, immunisation services were being delivered through 3400 static and outreach clinics nationwide. Outreach clinics provide 80% of immunisation services. Health surveillance assistants (HSAs), more than any other health cadre, deliver the EHP, including EPI at community level (see Chapter 6).

An EPI performance assessment made by researchers at the University of Malawi showed that the EPI has been both effective and equitable (Bowie et al. 2006). It has been the pride of the Malawian government for many years. Its efficiency has paid off in terms of external funding. GAVI requires 70% coverage as a criterion for providing health system support (see also Chapter 3). Based on demographic and health surveys (DHSs) from 1992 and 2000 the assessment shows that coverage is even high in districts with poor access to immunisation services. The Malawian health official blamed the measles outbreak on the tedious procurement procedures within the SWAp. But the reasons for an outbreak are multifaceted and complex.

Medical evidence: the measles vaccine

Unanticipated outbreaks of measles have been major setbacks to routine health care, overburdening an already weak system. Some argue that measles outbreaks can be anticipated, allowing countries and systems to plan their activities to control or avoid them. The interval between epidemic peaks is proportional to the number of susceptible individuals. If the immunisation rate is above 85%, the interval between peaks of disease can be 10 years, but if these levels of coverage are not reached, the interval can be as little as 3–4 years.

It is important to be aware that the coverage needed to eliminate different infections varies from one pathogen to another. The more infectious the disease the greater the need for high vaccine coverage. This model is based on the definition of basic reproductive rate that is defined as the average number of secondary infections produced when one infectious individual is introduced into a population of susceptible hosts. Infectious pathogens can be classified on a scale that allows the minimal vaccine coverage needed to eliminate the pathogen to be calculated. For instance, smallpox ($R0 = 2$–4) is less infectious than poliomyelitis ($R0$ 6–8), and the latter is less infectious than measles virus ($R0$ 16–18). Thus, measles is particularly difficult to eliminate since it needs very high vaccine coverage.

Studies from the Americas have shown that the elimination of measles demands more than the single vaccination dose that Malawi's EPI routinely provides. The optimism of elimination of measles has been achieved in Africa by administering a second dose of vaccine through supplementary immunisation days (campaigns). The SWAp had budgeted for such a campaign in 2012, just after Malawi suffered the outbreak.

The measles vaccine is safe, inexpensive, and effective when given to a child after measles antibodies acquired from the mother have disappeared

(Markowitz et al. 1990; Stephenson 2002). The important challenge for a successful measles control programme, however, is not only to reach and maintain high vaccination coverage but to achieve and maintain high immunity at the population level. The measles vaccine is 80% protective after a first dose and the immunogenicity is increased when administered correctly at the appropriate age. The latter is determined by precise concentration of infant maternal antibodies against measles. The concentration has to be low to offer protection but not enough to interfere with the attenuated live virus as it is an active component of the measles vaccine.

The concept of maternal antibodies and prevaccination protection are unfamiliar to many EPI managers, and the measles schedule is taken from global recommendations. To optimise the benefit of vaccination, studies for the detection of serum antibodies are important, but these are demanding and costly. This forces low-income countries, including Malawi, to base their choice of the optimal age for immunising children against measles on evidence from other countries.

In low-income countries, the intensity of exposure to measles virus and a more rapid decline in maternal antibodies put infants at risk of acquiring measles at a younger age, when the risk of mortality from measles is high (Aaby and Clements 1989). As a result, measles vaccine is given at 9 months of age in many tropical settings. This is contrary to high-income countries, where measles vaccine is given based on knowledge of the immune status of the infant through zero-surveillance (detection of the antibody type IgG against measles virus in the blood serum). Recognition of such problems and the successful measles elimination in the Americas has moved WHO to suggest the same strategy in Africa. Through a combination of approaches, including supplementary immunisation activities, improved surveillance and improved case management, measles morbidity and mortality have been reduced in some African countries (Otten et al. 2003), although complete measles elimination in Africa seems unlikely in the near future.

Malawi's measles crisis exemplifies the tensions between the advanced scientific knowledge of experts and the practical challenges of implementing a control programme.

Vaccine availability in Malawi

As early as 2007 Malawi's Minister of Health, Marjorie Ngaunje, lamented that the country would soon experience shortages of vaccines due to the lengthy procurement procedures (*Daily Times* 2007). In a high-level meeting for donors in the nation's capital, Lilongwe, she said that although the sector's SWAp programme had been a success, it also faced huge challenges, such as persistent stock outs of essential drugs. Lengthy procurement procedures not only affected timely procurement of drugs, but also medical supplies such as vaccines and treated mosquito nets (ITNs). As these complexities in procurement remained unresolved there were worries that the country would soon start to experience shortages of vaccines and ITNs (*Daily Times* 2007). Another area of concern, the Minister explained, was the delay in recruitment of additional HSAs, who play an important role in the delivery of the community component of the EHP, including HIV/AIDS interventions. This delay, she said, could have been avoided if all partners financing the SWAp pool fund were using one set of rules. The minister said she hoped the meeting would resolve such issues and avoid further delays in the implementation of interventions that would improve the health indicators.

Apparently the high-level meeting did not resolve the issues of concern. A recent evaluation of the SWAp undertaken by the UK Department for International Development (DfID) and the MoH in Malawi (2010) also raises some doubts as to the efficiency of the SWAp and its ability to deliver. The DfID explains Malawi's strong performance in health by pointing to the success of their EPI programme, but the question arises as to whether those gains are achieved because of, or in spite of, the SWAp. There are some suggestions, the report states, that the rate of improvement is in fact declining because the plan of action has been resource based and not needs based. The DfID also raised concern about the procurement procedures. Despite sustained support for the central medical store, little progress has been made. To the DfID, however, the problem is not the complexity of partners in the SWAp playing by different rules, as indicated by the minister. It is the unwillingness of the Malawi presidential office to contract in a whole new management or recruit new staff for key management posts in the central medical store. Delay in solving the issue was so important for the global fund that has contributed US$500 million to the SWAp since 2003 that it held back disbursement and caused stock outs of essential supplies of drugs. The Malawian government is responsible, through the SWAp, for providing all traditional vaccines and related logistics, but it does not control the funds for procurement.

The Malawi EPI manager argued that the reason for the EPI success was its verticality, and she was worried that integration into the SWAp would destroy the programme. A report from the MoH in 2004 raised a similar concern, fearing that sustainability of the EPI would be threatened as it would have to compete for resources within the SWAp (Malawi Ministry of Health 2004b). Although the EPI was then provided with its own prioritised 'budget line' the programme, in her opinion, nevertheless suffered from budgeting and procurement procedures that subjected it to politics both within the SWAp and between the SWAp and the Malawian government. Broader political issues played a role, however, since at that time the health system had almost collapsed. Because of concerns about human rights violations and economic mismanagement by Malawi's government, donors froze budgetary support and the Malawi EPI thus fell prey to politics and to donor conditionality of aid.

An earlier study by Gauri and Khaleghian (2002) is interesting in this regard. Their analysis of immunisation coverage concludes that national coverage rates are in general more a function of effective supply side than demand side effects. Their findings underscore the importance of the exchange of professional knowledge, the autonomy of public health managers, the quality of national institutions, and the involvement of international agencies in raising immunisation coverage rates (Gauri and Khaleghian 2002, p. 35). The closer the EPI to political priorities and disputes the more vulnerable it becomes. The point made by Gauri and Khaleghian, however, is that the reason low-income countries fail to deliver on high-priority interventions such as immunisation is because of lack of demand. This suggests 'that the organisational determinant of immunisation programmes might depend less on their effect on the way they promote or dampen demand of interest groups and households . . . and more on their direct effect on the action of political and bureaucratic elites' (Gauri and Khaleghian 2002, p. 3). Immunisation, in order to be effective, requires a centralised and vertical mode of intervention where it does not fall prey to other priorities (Gauri and Khaleghian 2002).

Governing child health in Malawi

In Malawi the EPI is integrated into the Maternal and Child Health programme. The EPI programme was organised vertically until the MoH adopted the SWAp in 2005. The academic literature has long been full of debates regarding which approach to delivery is the most effective, and the two positions differ both philosophically and practically (e.g. Banerji 1984; Rifkin and Walt 1986). Vertical methods are based on a short-term outlook that solves a defined health issue through application of specified measures. The rationale of the new political economy of the global health architecture is that vertical approaches compel more efficient and targeted investment without damaging national health systems. The objectives of these vertical interventions are set globally and tend to reflect global priorities. Horizontal services, on the other hand, reflecting the PHC philosophy of the Alma-Ata declaration, are carried out as a long-term process that seeks to tackle the roots of ill health. Horizontal services, generally publicly financed, refer to more integrated demand-driven and resource-sharing health services enhanced by the establishment of permanent institutional infrastructure (Mills 1983). The dichotomy between vertical and horizontal is not as rigid in practice as it may seem in theory (Mills 1983, 1972; Ooms et al. 2008). Instead of a rigid vertical–horizontal divide it is more accurate to think in terms of a continuum, with the global polio eradication campaign at one extreme. The EPI started out as a vertical intervention; in many countries it remains so in terms of financing, but is nevertheless integrated at the point of delivery. In many countries EPI is made part of the integrated management of childhood illness, that is, a systematic approach to children's health which focuses on the whole child. This means not only focusing on prevention of disease but also curative care.

The EPI manager in Malawi recognises that it is not either/or when explaining the efficiency of her programme. When we spoke to her in 2008 she put a lot of emphasis on the efforts of the EPI in making the programme acceptable to the people it was meant to serve. 'We work with the communities', she said, and 'we work with the communities through the chiefs'. The chief's role is crucial in Malawian governance. Through the Chiefs Act of 1967 traditional leaders are responsible for settling disputes, connecting citizens to district assemblies, acting as gate-keepers for their subjects, and championing local development. To go through the chiefs with a programme is to give it a political identity. Their role is critical because they can either facilitate or disrupt and delay development. Traditional leaders (chiefs) play an important role in mobilising communities for any activity, including health. During special health campaigns such as measles vaccination campaigns and child health days the HSA relays the message to the chief, who instructs his assistants to announce it to the villagers. Health announcements are also made by the chief's or HSA's representatives at funerals, in churches, and at every appropriate gathering. Health services provided during the child health days take place at the chief's place—under the tree where the village court also convenes.

Social anthropologists doing research in Malawi have shown how the institution of village headmen and chiefs has fostered village communities in which development is spoken of as the personal responsibility of each community member. It is a responsibility, not a right (Danielsen 2011; Eggen 2011; Englund 2006). Most citizens are in principle positive towards hospitals and biomedical measures, including vaccinations, and make great efforts to obtain them. The political legitimacy that is granted to the programmes through the support of the chiefs has had an enormous impact on vaccine demand. Vaccinations are regarded as a normal routine activity associated with child health. This concept of demand is close to what Streefland (1999, p. 159) refers to as social vaccine demand. According to the EPI manager, the success of the Malawian EPI programme was attributable to a combination of the two, a vertical supply chain that ensured priority and delivery of vaccines, and integration into politically functioning institutions at the point of delivery: characteristic of the more horizontal modes of delivery.

Malawi's policy-makers recognise the political nature of their health interventions. In their planning they are anxious to consider geographical disparities, poverty and its distribution, resource limitations, and sometimes also long-term programme sustainability. They are well aware of the political dimension of their decisions on how services are to be delivered. Malawi's EPI programme is visible to everyone through its integration in a familiar and trusted political institution. It is part of a system of national and local governance. The Malawian government did not want much change to their EPI programme, and with good reason. Why should they change one of the few popular, well-functioning, and trusted programmes in the country? Protecting the EPI could be a wise policy in the Malawi context.

The incentives driving donors within the SWAp, however, are quite different. Quick results are needed if political support for additional funding from their own constituencies is to be secured. Much depends on the strategic importance of the target group at that particular time: whether children, women or the poor. Vaccine procurement is a problem largely because of the complex auditing rules of the different donors, reflecting the demands of their individual constituencies. Arguably, this is part of the game, but it is problematic when the accountability is structured so as to favour upwards accountability to donors rather than to the people the programme is meant to serve. In Malawi's measles outbreak this tension between the two accountability structures was made very apparent.

Facilitating childhood vaccination in India

Childhood immunisation has been an important part of maternal and childhood services in India since the 1940s, although coverage has always varied considerably across states, between rural and urban areas, and between genders.

In 1992, India's UIP became a part of the Child Survival and Safe Motherhood (CSSM) Programme and in 1997 an important component of the Reproductive and Child Health (RCH) Programme. The cold chain was strengthened, and training programmes were launched throughout the country. Intensified polio eradication activities were started in 1995–96 under the Polio Eradication Programme, beginning with NIDs and active surveillance for acute flaccid paralysis (AFP). The Polio Eradication Programme was set up with the assistance of the National Polio Surveillance Project.

Until 2004 India's public spending on health was amongst the lowest in the world, at less than 1% of gross domestic product. WHO's national health profile for India from 2002 stated that India compared unfavourably even with low-income countries with regard to human resources, particularly in rural areas (World Health Organization 2002). Notably, there was a critical shortage of health personnel in the government institutions that provided health care to the poorest segments of the population. While several initiatives have been taken to strengthen human resource management, some systemic issues remain unresolved, such as low morale and uncommitted staff owing to poor remuneration, and seniority-based promotion disregarding suitability and merit (India National Health System Profile).

India's current health policy has its origins in the nation-building activities that occurred during independence in 1947. The Government of India's *Report on the Health Survey and Development Committee*, referred to as the Bhore Committee Report (Peters et al. 2002) saw the nation's poor health as caused by unsanitary conditions, defective nutrition, inadequate health institutions, and lack of health education. The report provided comprehensive recommendations that included putting health workers on the public pay roll, limiting the need for private practitioners, a clear emphasis on preventive methods, and, importantly, a new infrastructure plan—a three-tier healthcare system at district level to provide both preventive and curative health care. Although many of the recommendations of the Bhore report were never implemented, it is seen as the foundation for the health reforms that followed. Notably, the Bhore Committee laid down the principle that access to primary health care is a fundamental right and established primary health care as a foundation for the national healthcare system.

Inspired by both the Bhore report and the Alma-Ata Declaration (WHO/UNICEF 1978) the National Health Policy of 1983 reinforced, in rhetoric, the establishment of a public health service system based on the foundation of a decentralised public primary healthcare system. In theory the three-tier system should provide health care to all rural inhabitants. At the lowest level, PHCs were designed to provide basic medical care, disease prevention, and health promotion education. The next tier, subcentres, were intended to provide public health services. A top tier of community centres and district hospitals offered specialist services. By the end of 1980 an extensive health service infrastructure had been developed and a substantial number of health workers trained. In the 10-year period 1980–1990, the number of PHCs almost quadrupled (from 5500 to 20, 536) and the number of doctors increased by more than 100,000 (Quader 2000).

Constitutionally, health care in India is largely the responsibility of the provincial states. In general, almost 90% of public expenditure comes through the state budget. The central government is in charge of defining policies and providing national strategic frameworks. Central funding consists of specific-purpose grants for public health (nutrition, water supply, and sanitation), family planning, and disease control programmes, which fall under what is referred to as a 'minimum need programme' (Purohit 2001). In practice, states struggled to maintain and administer the system, and became over time more and more dependent on central government for both technical and financial resources (Peter et al. 2002). The promise of India's first national health policy, of building a vast health infrastructure for primary health care and closely coordinated health services, did not evolve into an integrated system. Rather, the health system came to consist of a myriad of vertical health programmes operating in near-isolation from the formal health system, including family planning programmes, polio eradication efforts, and various vaccination campaigns (Das Gupta 2005). Various ministries administered matters that directly affected population health, with no coordinating mechanism among them. Similarly, there was a division between the national and the state level within the health sector itself. Whereas the national health authorities took care of national health priorities formulated as specific vertical programmes, the individual states catered for the maintenance of the health system. For the UPI this implied that the government procured vaccines and set coverage targets, whereas the individual state maintained the cold chain.

In the early 1990s India adopted the policy of structural adjustment, a process that involved liberalisation of the economy and reduction of the budgetary deficit. A consequence was that government expenditure on social sectors, including health, was severely cut. In this period the central component of public health and disease control programmes grant was rigorously curtailed. Central funds for disease control fell from 41.47 to 18.50% in this period, a cut which had the most pronounced effect on the poorer states (Purohit 2001, pp. 87–88). The achievements of the health reform of 1983 suffered a severe setback.

In the last few years the Indian government has set about correcting for these setbacks and things have changed. According to World Bank statistics, per capita, health expenditure in India increased from US$30 to 54 during the period 2005–2010. This is double the health expenditure per capita of Malawi (US$16–26 per capita) The main reason in India for this rise in expenditure was the launch of the NRHM, the reform system introduced in April 2005. The NRHM is an attempt at an integrated approach to address essential health care in rural areas that encompasses integration of earlier vertical interventions into routine horizontal primary health care within an overarching health plan. The most substantial investment of the NRHM has been the new health cadre, the ASHA, a community health mobiliser recruited from and situated within her own community. There is one ASHA per 1000 people.

When NRHM was launched it was explained in terms of human rights and universal access to health care. Since independence, inequality has been a stated concern of the Indian government. In the 1940s the first Indian Prime Minister, Jawaharlal Nehru, saw the state as provider, protector, and promoter—responsible for ensuring that all Indian citizens, men and women, would enjoy equal rights to growth and access to the health services (Government of India Planning Commission 1952, p. 29, quoted in Corbridge et al. 2005, p. 55). At the same time Nehru acknowledged that the country's traditional systems of class and caste represented a major challenge to equal rights for all. When launched, the NRHM was therefore presented as a belated fulfilment of early post-independence promises. Healthcare seekers were encouraged to speak up on their own account and to hold government health institutions accountable for the services they provided. This agenda mobilised a concept of empowerment that emphasises individual self-worth and the realisation of individual potential in the face of long-standing inequalities in access to education and care. The key point was that people should put themselves in the position of a customer and demand that the services they received were of good quality (Corbridge et al. 2005, p. 78).

As we have seen, the health MDGs provide national health policy-makers with comprehensive and time-bound goals, targets, and indicators, and, as such, a powerful framework for health priorities. India accounts for 21% of global deaths of children under 5 years of age. Heavy pressure was therefore put on India to adopt the MDG framework and reduce child mortality by a third by 2015. The Government of India adopted ambitious targets that are in line with, and sometimes even more ambitious than, the MDGs. For MDG4 India adopted the target and has shown some progress (2.6 point reduction rate), but the current rate of progress is, according to UNICEF, not sufficient to meet the target by 2015. In order for that to happen there should be a minimum 7.6 point reduction (UNICEF SOWC 2008). The percentage of children under 1 year of age immunised against measles is used as an indicator of child health. According to the Third National Family Health Survey (NFHS-3), the percentage of children aged between 12 and 23 months who had received a measles vaccination by 12 months of age was reported to be only 48.4%, while the total percentage was found to be 58.8% (NFHS-3). The 11th Five-Year Strategic Plan has set reduction of the infant mortality rate to 28/1000 live births as a goal (Government of India 2008). The government is directing intensive efforts to improvement of child health, notably the interventions under the RCH Programme. These address a wide range of interventions against the leading causes of childhood morbidity and mortality: acute respiratory infections, diarrhoea, malaria, measles, and malnutrition.

Providing child healthcare under the NRHM

Central to the child health strategy is the child health card: a token not only of child health management but also of citizenship. The child health card carries clear messages on entitlements to services, rights, and duties. It explains the minimum package of entitlements (what one may expect from the state) and the corresponding duties (what one should do as a responsible citizen). It can be seen as a tool for the management of children's health at the interface between state and the child's care-givers.

The child health card was originally developed by WHO. At the outset it was only a vaccination card under the EPI, but as child health management developed in relation to the immunisation schedule it has come to include a growth chart and information about general child health management. With the renewed focus on MDGs and the integration of MDG4 and MDG5 into maternal and child health, the card includes information and entitlements relating to both pre- and antenatal care, and has become one of the central tools used in health education. The child health card can assist healthcare providers to offer high-quality care to infants and children. Furthermore, it provides the child's parents or guardians with information to help them look after the child properly. It thus has multiple purposes: it can be used as evidence for health worker performance (as discussed in Chapter 6), for monitoring child care management by parents and guardians, and as a basis for monitoring children's development at the population level. In this sense it could be used to assess the overall effects of the government's child health services (see Figure 5.3).

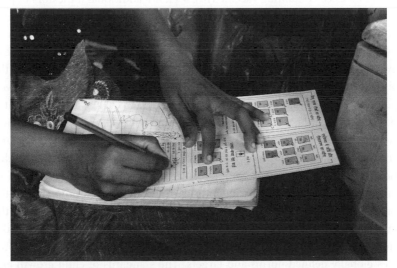

Fig. 5.3 The health card and vaccine registration.
Photo: Courtesy of Dagrun Kyte Gjøstein.

The health card

In 2006 WHO published new international growth standards: curves characterising the normal growth of children aged 0 to 59 months. The charts were based on studies of healthy populations in each of six countries (Brazil, Ghana, India, Norway, Oman and the USA), selected to reduce the impact of environmental variation. The study found remarkable similarity in early childhood growth patterns and a universal growth chart was crafted and included in the child health card. Indian government experts questioned the universal validity of the WHO's new growth chart. Although sceptical, the Indian Academy of Paediatricians approved it, but only because India was one of the six countries in the WHO study, and only until norms specific to the Indian population have been developed.

The child health card is a key tool in generating reliable data. Conventionally coverage on routine immunisation activities is measured by dividing the number of doses distributed by the size of the target population. This method leads to coverage estimates that are sometimes impossible (e.g. vaccination of 102% of the target population). Administrative coverage estimates derived like this are reported annually to WHO and UNICEF. Using these, plus special surveys and other published and unpublished data, WHO and UNICEF derive national estimates of vaccination coverage through a country-by-country review of the best available data. DTP3 coverage by age 12 months serves as the primary indicator of immunisation programme performance, although coverage with other recommended vaccines, including the third dose of polio vaccine and the first dose of measles-containing vaccine (MCV1), are additional indicators of programme strength. The DHS project is responsible for collecting and disseminating accurate, nationally representative data on health and population in developing countries. These are widely referred to as the most reliable source of coverage data. DHS methodology is based on the information given on the child heath card. Since this card is an attempt at a universal health card developed by WHO in collaboration UNICEF, USAID, UNAIDS, and UNFPA it is not subject to national politics. But here again India with its strong statistical resources has developed its own survey, the NFHS, a large-scale, multi-round survey conducted in a representative sample of households throughout India. The child health card gives an interesting insight into the distribution of managerial and political authority. In brief, the planning is top-down, and the dominant mechanisms for accountability are upwards, almost by-passing the national government, to global and multilateral institutions. The child health card is framed within a universal concept of the body and the person, and provides globally defined norms and targets. The standards of child growth and development are established not in an MoH but globally, and based on children's development under optimal conditions. The question arises whether the use of universal standards, such as optimal growth for children, is making 'the perfect the enemy of the good'. In an article from 2007 Clemens et al. raise the question in relation to the universal MDG goals as they relate to individual countries. Is it just, they ask, to work with similar indicators representing the efforts of countries with:

> vast natural resources alongside those with none, countries in conflict and in peace; donor darlings and global pariahs; those with heightened access to natural resources and those without; communist and capitalist; autocratic and democratic, high saving and low savings; those with ready access to foreign investment and those without, those infested with disease and those in more salubrious climes (Clemens et al. 2007, p. 746).

It is debatable where India features in this picture, combining as it does impressive economic growth and wealth creation with stagnation in key social indicators. India certainly faces enormous health challenges and has embarked on comprehensive and challenging health interventions—and in a society that is extremely heterogeneous in terms of class, caste, ethnicity, and religion. In line with the MDG targets, India does set priorities and support immunisation, family planning and facility based births, with incentives for health workers. But when the multipurpose health card is not only tracking the health of children and mothers but also the performance of care takers, health workers, and states, it becomes problematic. When performance is linked to incentives and salaries it is, as will be shown in Chapter 6, distorting not only numbers indicating health status and performance, but also priorities. Indicators are powerful in this respect and narrow the vision of a complex and comprehensive intervention such as the NRHM was, and still is, intended to be. The NRHM gives high priority to immunisation and spends more than US$500 million every year in immunising children against vaccine-preventable diseases. Their main tool in increasing immunisation coverage is the village health-worker ASHA and her role in community mobilisation.

Community mobilisation

The revival of the community health worker, an influential idea in international public health in the 1980s, represents what Shaw and Martin (2000) refer to as a 'recycling of community' in contemporary health interventions. This is an informative observation on Indian state health policies. Within notions of community work, citizenship is asserted as a formally ascribed political status and a collective asserted political practice (Nordfeldt and Roalkvam 2010). Both the citizen and the community should, under the NRHM, determine their own needs and become full partners in the decision-making process. Thus village health committees are established alongside and with the same structure as the Panchayati. The Panchayati is a three-tier system within the state with elected bodies from villages helping ensure democratic participation and public anchoring of development and health programmes. This is thus a governance structure comparable with the institutions of chief and headman in Malawi. Importantly, the chief in Malawi is not an elected representative—in fact the institution of chief is contested. However the village headman, like the village health committee in India, is responsible for developing a village health plan, for health assessments and priorities, for creating awareness of health services and entitlements, and for overseeing the work of village health workers such as the ASHA and the auxiliary nurse midwife (ANM), and in the case of Malawi the HSAs.

The village health committee is part of the Indian government's efforts at decentralising health policy and planning, often referred to as an attempt at bringing control closer to the people, or as engaging the public in the attempt to improve health and well-being. The intention is that investment in health should be controlled by the people and reflect the needs of the people. The term 'demand side' appears thus with increased frequency in pro-poor health planning and policy. The main drivers behind the increased interest in demand are located in the economic and institutional crisis and transformations of national health sectors: increasing marketisation and provider pluralism, and the collapse, in many countries, of public sector services and governance. The idea, it seems, is that the variety and quality of care should expand in response to demand from the people. NRHM focuses explicitly on decentralisation and enhancing demand by revitalising local political institutions such as Panchayati, and the innovative use of incentives for health seekers and health workers in public health facilities. There is increasing recognition of the way national and subnational inequalities affect health outcomes. That the poor that NRHM tries to reach have critical and negative experiences of the health services is also increasingly recognised. Underutilisation of health services has therefore been seen as one of the major challenges. The determinants of this are complex and encompass not only cost factors but also indifferent treatment, rude behaviour from providers, gender barriers within the household, and a host of other cultural and social constraints. Individuals and households face an unregulated environment in which the boundaries between public and private become increasingly blurred. They also face this market from a position of information inequality.

Contextual factors such as these have spurred efforts at mobilising the demand side in order to achieve health gains. There is considerable debate and experimentation on ways to reduce out-of-pocket expenditure, and to improve the quality and responsiveness of public services. The argument has been that understanding and working with the demand side is the key to both objectives. This has again led to two main demand-side concerns. One is understanding health-seeking behaviour and patterns of utilisation with a view either to changing them or better catering for them. The second is to find ways of harnessing the demand side to press for improving the responsiveness of the supply side. The ASHAs in India are trained to work as a bridge, spanning the gap between the local community and the public health system to secure community ownership through various intersectoral convergence mechanisms under the NRHM. The importance of village health workers will be discussed further in Chapter 6.

Health systems and policies in context

Immunisation programmes and disease control do not operate as free-standing activities but form part of the variety of health packages delivered through national health systems. According to WHO, health systems have three fundamental objectives: improve the health of the population they serve, respond to people's expectations, and provide financial protection against the costs of ill health (World Health Organization 2000). A health system, again according to WHO, is defined by the organisations, people, and actions whose primary intent is to promote, restore or maintain health. This includes efforts to influence determinants of health as well as more direct health-improving activities. Ideally a health system ensures the provision of preventive, curative, rehabilitative, and other public health services, as well as the building up of the necessary pool of financial, physical, and human resources (Mills et al. 2007). To date most attempts at strengthening health systems in developing countries have been based on technical approaches informed by burden of disease, cost-effectiveness analysis, and the results of clinical trials (Byskov et al. 2009). Technical approaches, important as they are, leave out the sociocultural aspects of health systems. Health system functioning also depends on relationships between individuals, and between individuals and social systems. Marchal et al. see health systems as complex and open systems, drawing resources from their environment and responsive to the people and communities they serve (Marchal et al. 2009, p. 4). In cost-effectiveness terms immunisation is one of public health's 'best buys', but vaccines are not necessarily a response to what people feel they need. Bisht and Coutinho (2000) describe how, during a polio boycott in northern India, vaccination was seen by the local communities as something inflicted on them by force, when what they wanted was clean water, sanitation, better housing, and schools. As a minority Muslim community within a majority Hindu state everything the government did or did not do was informed by and understood within this context. Public health services are profoundly important sites where citizens and state interact (Nordfeldt and Roalkvam 2010).

Trust in a health system is influenced not only by the quality of the services offered, but also by communities' relations to the government, by accountability, fairness, and a range of other values. Low immunisation coverage can be due to a lack of trust in the system and its representatives. For example, Roalkvam has shown how India's population control campaign in the 1970s resulted in local communities losing trust in public facilities. In the 1970s, concerns about India's rapidly growing population led to vigorous birth-control campaigns that people resisted on both economic and religious grounds. Because of the heavy resistance, the Indian government initiated a sterilisation campaign, at first voluntary but later also enforced—at times with brute force. Memories of these procedures have become part of a common attitude towards governmental facilities (Nordfeldt and Roalkvam 2010; Roalkvam 2012).

Contemporary health systems are multifaceted and deeply political, and conceal dynamic relationships between the people and institutions that constitute them. India, for example, has seen a steady migration of skilled personnel from government to the private sector institutions, and abroad. In many countries in Africa mobility of skilled personnel has resulted in a virtual collapse of the delivery system (Marchal et al. 2009, p. 63).

We began this chapter by referring to billboards advertising presidential health messages, and we continued with a discussion of cold-chain maintenance, routine immunisation, and the management of outbreaks—all ways in which the state is engaged with the management of life and by which it makes itself visible to its citizens. The prevailing focus on technical issues, we suggested, draws attention away from the political nature of justice and equitable participation. Whereas global initiatives as well as governments emphasise citizens as rights bearers in political rhetoric, they appear rather as units of population in policies, health science, and in the setting of priorities and interventions. Soysal (1994) has a compelling argument which has, at its centre, the assertion that a new and more universal concept of citizenship is unfolding—one whose organising and legitimating principle is based on universal embodiment and personhood rather than on national belonging (Soysal 1994, p. 1). In other words, it is similarities that are emphasised not differences. The context of this shift is the development of international law, the UN system, global civil society, and human rights. The language of human rights challenges the idea that states are sovereign in relation to their citizens. However, even though globalisation has altered the context within which states govern, it is the state that remains the primary context for the individual citizen. Rights and responsibilities are still exercised mainly at the level of the state. Similarly, as we have seen, multilateral organisations and new global health initiatives rely on states for the enactment of their health initiatives.

We have seen above how responses to an epidemic mirror the functioning of political systems. We have argued that public health and healthcare delivery are crucial, and that the health and welfare of people is an index not only of the economic progress of nations but also of the legitimacy of their governments. In contemporary discourse the legitimacy of governments is said to lie in their performance—the provision of financial assistance, public services, and other benefits to their people. States needs something to do. In an era of rapid globalisation Sen (1999) set out to make development relevant in a new context of market-oriented policies as opposed to state-oriented development. The basic idea was to create space for state-based development without ignoring the logic of the market. The state, he argued, should be involved in areas where market failure was more evident rather than in production of marketable commodities. States should concentrate on health and education, aiming to fashion people-centred policies and pro-poor growth. It was an attempt to prevent the state being pushed into oblivion when subjected to the forces of globalisation and market liberalisation. The success of the Malawi EPI indicates that ownership, so frequent a word in development texts, is not an optional extra for aid delivery. Nor is health governance (or 'political will') something to be engineered by donors; rather it is fundamentally about existing institutions, power, and politics, and the exercise of entitlements in society. Governance is both practised and experienced. This fact may also explain its failures. A conventional conception of decentralisation comprises national projects like the NRHM in India or the EPI in Malawi that work outwards and downwards through the formal structures and procedures of local government; the institution of chiefs and village head men, or the village Panchayati or health committees. However, with their technocratic rules, procedures, and incentives even decentralised systems like the NRHM work with an accountability structure upward to central government, state, donors, and global health initiatives, rather than downward to the people.

The MDGs challenge the political identity of the state as they are not seen as responsible for the interventions that follow in their wake. Nor, it may be argued, are the MDG priorities what people themselves feel that they need, but rather a global perspective imposed on national governments and emanating from a particular global vision of the world (Brada 2011). We may ask if we are witnessing new practices of government and forms of politics. According to

Fergusson and Gupta (2002), in popular state discourse two images are dominant: *verticality* and *encompassment*. Verticality refers to the notion that the state is an institution in some sense above civil society, community, and the family. Thus state planning is naturally top-down and state efforts are efforts to control and plan from above. Does this imply also an image of political hierarchy, power, and authority? The state or global community is 'somewhere up there' operating at a 'higher level', but the state is made effective and authoritative by its performance, i.e. how the state makes itself visible to its people (Fergusson and Gupta 2002). Donors, as we have seen (in Chapter 3), have focused on governance through a much-restricted lens—the technical management of government resources and effective implementation of different sector policies. Whereas global vaccine initiatives contribute to the health agenda by crafting specific innovations and providing evidence in support of these interventions, governments remain primarily responsible for building and maintaining the infrastructure that facilitates the flow of these innovations. Moreover the MDG health goals cover only a small share of the total burden of disease within a country. Improving health is an inherently political process that cannot be divorced from specific economic, social, and cultural contexts.

Citizenship implies a political community if it is to have meaning. Malawians capture this tight relation between the state and citizens in the management of health when they refer to the immunisation card as a 'health passport'. The health card is not only an indicator of a child's immunisation status, it is also a concrete expression of citizenship, and the rights and obligations that entails. Citizenship is a dynamic identity. It defies a simple static definition that can be applied to all countries at all times. Citizenship is inherently contested and contingent, reflecting a particular set of relationships and governance found within any society.

Conclusions

Immunisation programmes do not operate as free-standing activities but are part of the variety of health packages delivered through national health systems. We have argued that the health system is a core social institution that structures relations between citizens and the state. This is especially apparent in a situation of a pandemic outbreak, when governments need to be visible and proactive; their political legitimacy is at stake. We have argued that in governing health the state (most notably in poor countries) has changed from being the central, dominating source of authority within a defined territory to becoming an activator or coordinator of the activities of external actors and

institutions. In the era of the health MDG governments are required to perform on the MDG targets, and the policies and tools for achieving them are
largely externally defined. Indicators play a powerful role in this situation; they
narrow the vision of a complex and comprehensive national intervention such
as the NRHM in India, or distort well-functioning programmes like the Malawi EPI. Targets and indicators are important for donors and their constituency,
but often of less value to individual countries that are pursuing broader and
longer term reforms. The Malawi EPI and the Indian NRHM, despite their differences, both make a sincere attempt at community participation. Community participation in decision-making planning and action is referred to as a
human right, and through the institution of the chiefs in Malawi or the Indian
Panchayati health interventions are linked to formal and recognised governance structures. It is increasingly argued that new styles and structures of governance are needed, such that instead of being passive recipients of services
provided, as a target population, people enjoy genuine participation—as citizens. On the other hand, health is now not only part of a country's national but
also its foreign policy portfolio. How these developments are to be reconciled
remains to be seen.

Chapter 6

'Immunisation is good for your children': local immunisation practices in India and Malawi

Arima Mishra, Rune Flikke, Cecilie Nordfeldt, and Lot Nyirenda

Introduction

In this chapter we turn to immunisation practices at the interface between the national health systems of India and Malawi and local communities. It is here, at the local level, that the flow of technology (vaccine) reaches its end users—the children—thus linking the global technology to the individual body. Moreover what happens at the local level generates the raw data on immunisation 'coverage' which are used as measures of the success of immunisation programmes. It is also at this interface that narratives of compliance, resistance, and adherence are produced. In approaching the interface, as anthropologists, we follow the steps introduced in Chapter 2: (a) where is it (b) who is involved and (c) what goes on here?

The first step leads us to the local sites at which vaccines are delivered to children in India and Malawi. National governments deploy a variety of healthcare delivery structures and personnel to take vaccines to the local level. Often different modes of delivery are combined; for instance both fixed health centres and periodic immunisation days for specific vaccines may be used. In India, for example, we find fixed health centres (some public and some private), national and subnational immunisation days (mostly for polio), catch-up campaigns for immunisation (especially against measles), and routine immunisation days. The last are organised in fixed rural health centres and in outreach clinics in villages, under the jurisdiction of the health centres. In Malawi, similarly, vaccines are delivered on a regular basis in fixed health units run by the government, by CHAM, and by private institutions. Hospitals and health centres organise outreach clinic services, which reach out to rural and isolated communities. At designated periods during the year Malawi's EPI arranges NIDs, which are special immunisation campaigns supporting global goals. NIDs in Malawi target measles, polio, and vitamin A supplementation, while in India they usually focus on polio. Of all these different mechanisms for vaccine delivery we chose to focus on two: on routine immunisation days (also known as mother–child health and nutrition days) in India, and on outreach clinics in Malawi. For both India and Malawi, where 70% and 80% (respectively) of the population lives in rural areas, these two sites, specifically designed to reach children living in remote areas, are crucial. Unlike periodic campaigns, vaccination at these two sites occurs regularly (a fixed day every month) and involves continuous interactions between the state health personnel responsible for managing and administering the vaccines and the local community. Due to the regularity of the event, these sites are stable, observable locations in which we could study the dynamics of the interactions and social processes leading to immunisation outcomes. Like the outreach clinics in Malawi, routine immunisation days in the two study states of Orissa and Rajasthan in India are conducted through outreach sessions in the villages.

Who is present at these sites? The first, most visible, actors are the village level health workers who represent the state. In Malawi these are the HSAs; in India a multilayered set of health workers are involved: ASHAs, ANMs, and AWWs. The ASHAs were added to the state health bureaucracy in 2005. They are responsible for mobilising the community to access public health services, particularly immunisation, hospital birth, and antenatal care services. They are not paid a regular salary but on the basis of performance. An ASHA should have 8 years of schooling and be a married woman living in the village in which she operates. One ASHA is appointed for every 1000 people. They receive about 3 weeks of training spread over a period of 5 years. While the ASHAs are designated by name as community activists, they are, as we will see later, treated very much as government workers. The ANMs are above the ASHAs in the health bureaucracy and additionally exercise authority over the ASHAs through having been trained to provide curative services for minor ailments and administer vaccines. An ANM will generally have 18 months of training. Unlike the ASHAs, the ANMs have been a part of the health bureaucracy and primary health care since the 1950s. However, their roles have changed over time, and their responsibilities have been extended to include maternal and child health services, family planning services, nutrition and health education, immunisation, and the treatment of minor ailments (Malik 2009). The ANMs are permanent salaried government employees, paid satisfactory wages by current standards (approximately 10,000 rupees or US$180). Unlike the ASHAs, ANMs do not reside in the villages that they serve (four or five villages are under the jurisdiction of one ANM). The ANM travels to these villages on different days, immunisation day being the most important one. An ANM is responsible for a health subcentre (the lowest health centre in the hierarchy of health institutions that connect the local villages to the national health system) covering a population of around 5000. The AWWs are also women workers recruited from the village to act as a bridge between the formal health system and the community. They work at the intersection between the health and education needs of small children and the healthcare needs of mothers. An AWW is a locally recruited, monthly salaried teacher of an Anganwadi centre organised by the Department of Women and Child Development. At these centres, breastfeeding mothers and children between birth and 5 years are given supplementary food, and pre-school activities are arranged for children between 3 and 4 years. An AWW receives a monthly salary well below that of an ANM (2000 rupees or US$36). In Rajasthan, the ASHA is employed at the Anganwadi Centre in parallel with her duties to the health department, for which she receives an almost symbolic monthly payment (1000 rupees or US$18). Apart from this variety of health workers, we also found parents, their children, and extended kin networks, including grandparents, other relatives, and neighbours at our site. Occasionally in India there might also be village-level schoolteachers and local NGO employees (specifically for special campaigns like World Hand-Washing Day and World Population Day).

In Malawi, it is the HSAs that link the formal health system with communities. Their history dates back to the 1960s, when they were recruited as smallpox vaccinators. Following a cholera outbreak in the 1970s, the smallpox vaccinators were appointed as cholera assistants. The MoH retained the cholera assistants, now renamed HSAs, in the early 1980s (Kadzandira and Chilowa 2001), but it was not until 1995 that HSAs were formally incorporated into the MoH hierarchy, working in non-established posts until 2011, when their positions were established (Hermann et al. 2009; Nyirenda and Flikke 2012). They are centrally recruited by the MoH and posted to their duty stations after undergoing 10 weeks of training (Hermann et al. 2009). The monthly salaries of the HSAs during our fieldwork in 2010 ranged from 9900 kwacha (US$64) to about 13,000 kwacha (US$84) for senior HSAs. Before 2006, there were around 5000 HSAs in Malawi, the majority of whom had 2 or 4 years of secondary education, with a very few having only primary school qualifications. In 2006, 6000 HSAs with a 4-year secondary education certificate were recruited with support from the Global Fund to fight AIDS, tuberculosis and malaria (Katsulukuta 2010). There is supposed to be one HSA per 1000 population, although as of 2010 the actual ratio was 1:1200 (Katsulukuta 2010). The HSAs, who are supposed to reside within their communities, have responsibility for three to seven villages depending on the population and the size of the areas. In reality, many HSAs do not reside within the communities where they work. Many explain this by referring to a lack of adequate accommodation. The HSAs are supervised by environmental health officers, who have degree qualifications in environmental health and are based at the district hospitals.

Like the ANMs in India, HSAs are also involved in various activities in addition to immunisation; the number of tasks added over the years is so extensive that the majority of our HSA informants had difficulties listing all the activities in their job description (Alfsen 2011). All HSAs conduct immunisation, growth monitoring, disease investigation, water and sanitation and health education, and community mobilisation. They also deliver services during child health days. Immunisation has always been one of their core tasks, and HSAs are said to deliver more than 60% of EPI services. In our study districts, almost all immunisation activities we observed were indeed carried out by HSAs, and it is they who provide regular immunisation services in the hard-to-reach areas. Selected HSAs deliver services such as HIV counselling and testing, family planning, treatment of minor/uncomplicated illnesses such as malaria, pneumonia and diarrhoea, and carry out home visits for neonatal care referrals (Kadzandira and Chilowa 2001; Katsulukuta 2010; Alfsen 2011, p. 109ff).

What happens at these sites? As noted earlier, they are the primary source of evidence on 'immunisation coverage'. It is the numbers produced here that give rise to national success stories such as that of Malawi, and to India's more chequered story (reflecting major inter-regional variations). What does high coverage in Malawi then imply and what does the relatively low and uneven coverage among different regions and ethnic groups in Rajasthan and Orissa tell us about the vaccination behaviour of the communities involved? How should we understand 'vaccination coverage' data? In public health discourse the term is widely used as a proxy indicator for vaccine demand. Anthropologists, on the other hand, have pointed out the limitations of such indicators, and suggested that coverage data represent an unreliable construction that tells little of the vaccination behaviour of people (Nichter 1995; Greenough 1995; Streefland et al. 1999; Fairhead et al. 2004; Leach and Fairhead 2005). Compliance with vaccination regimes, they suggest, is not an individual decision and nor is it determined by the merits of the vaccine technology alone. Vaccination decisions have to be understood in terms of a larger context, which some anthropologists refer to as the 'local vaccination culture' (Streefland 1995; Streefland et al. 1999; Leach and Fairhead 2005). This notion of culture links the variation in demand to the vaccination's compatibility with existing knowledge, aetiologies, and perceptions of disease, with specific sociocultural-political contexts, and with the interactions between people and healthcare providers that take place there. Importantly, the concept of local vaccination culture critiques the stereotypical understanding in health promotion approaches, where 'culture' is often used to denote public ignorance of the merits of vaccines. Empirical studies reveal the complexity of vaccination practices and the difficulty of predicting them on the basis of, for example, the educational level of mothers or the adequacy of the vaccine supply (Bisht and Coutinho 2000; Samuelsen 2001; Serquina-Ramiro et al. 2001; Fairhead, Leach and Small 2004; Babalola and Lawan 2009).

High or low coverage in itself tells us little about compliance, adherence, or resistance. Only through examining national–local interfaces at specific sites of vaccine delivery can we understand how immunisation outcomes emerge. The processes of reinterpretation out of which they emerge differ from site to site. They reflect the interplay of a host of factors: the relationships between health workers and parents, communication strategies, the ways in which vaccination is linked to (and may be a condition for accessing) other health services, social relations within and amongst the community, and—not least—trust in individual health workers, in public health services, and in the technology itself.

Study sites

In order to explore these processes and relationships we carried out 6 months of ethnographic fieldwork in two states in India (focusing specifically on one district in each of these states) and in two districts in Malawi. The locations of the places at which we did our fieldwork are shown in Figures 6.1 and 6.2. In the course of the 6 months we spent at each site we observed immunisation days and other community events, including child protection rituals and healing sessions. We also conducted in-depth interviews with villagers, health workers, and officials at block- and district-level health centres. The Malawian districts were chosen on the basis of their differential performance according to coverage data provided by EPI. On this basis, one of our sites (Dowa) was a better performing district than the other (Thyolo). Both the Indian states in which we did our fieldwork (Orissa and Rajasthan) have relatively low coverage. However, we chose to focus on relatively well-performing communities in each state, both in order to have something to observe and to see what actually works when it works.

While Rajasthan and Orissa are both states in the federation of India and their health systems have been built up along similar lines, their histories and population characteristics differ from one to the other, as do many cultural traits. This has important implications for the way negotiations over immunisation play out. The hot and dry plains of the western Indian state of Rajasthan lie close to the national capital of Delhi. Rajasthan is presently the largest Indian state, with

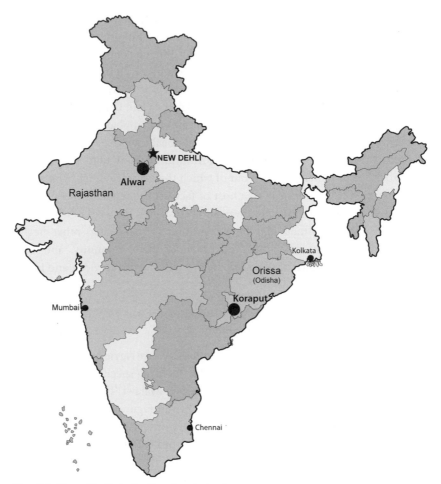

Fig. 6.1 Map of India indicating the study sites.
Map adapted from Rajeshodayanchal at ml.wikipedia.org (CC BY-SA 3.0).

342,240 km^2 or 10.4% of the total area of the country. According to the 2011 census the population is 68 million, of which nearly 90% is Hindu. Muslims, 8% of the population, are the largest minority (Census of India 2011). Jains—the merchants and traders from Rajasthan—also constitute a significant presence. Scheduled castes (SC) and Scheduled tribes (ST) form about 70% and 12%, respectively, of the state population. Previously Rajasthan was divided into many princely states. These states had seen shifting rulers, including Muslim, Moghuls, and later Hindu kings, who allied with the British in different ways during colonial times. The population traditionally survived from a variety of interconnected

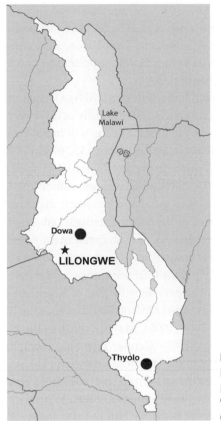
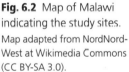

Fig. 6.2 Map of Malawi indicating the study sites. Map adapted from NordNord-West at Wikimedia Commons (CC BY-SA 3.0).

and caste-stratified forms of employment, including cattle herding, trade, military or court services, religious services, and agriculture. Today, Rajasthan is a conglomerate of different ethnic, religious, caste, and class groups. This is reflected in the composition in the densely populated areas of our fieldwork sites where even relatively small villages could be composed of Hindus, Muslims, indigenous people called 'tribal', and high and low castes and classes. Social life is characterised by complex patterns of segmentation and hierarchies along ethnic, caste, and class lines. Rajasthan lags behind the rest of the country in terms of key health indicators. Its maternal mortality ratio (445/100,000) is one of the highest in the country, whilst the infant mortality rate in rural Rajasthan (69/1000) is the fifth highest in India. The female literacy rate (43.9%) is far lower than the country figure of 53.7%. In terms of immunisation coverage, Rajasthan is considered as a low-performing state in India, with only 48.7% of eligible children being fully immunised (DLHS 3 2007–2008). For the major vaccines, the percentages for BCG, DPT3, polio 3, and measles are 82.6%, 55.6%, 63.9% and 67.3%, respectively (DLHS 3 2007–2008). A community-based, cross-sectional survey undertaken in the study district in Rajasthan shows the percentage of fully immunised children to be only 28.9% (Jain et al. 2006).

Orissa, at the eastern edge of India, is dominated by a large number of indigenous (or 'tribal') populations, concentrated mostly in the western and southern parts of the state. According to the latest census of India, the population of Orissa state is 42 million. It has an area of about 155,707 km^2. Geographically Orissa can be divided into three distinctive regions: the coastal plains, the middle mountainous country, and the plateaux and rolling uplands. This geographical division corresponds to social and economic divisions as well, with coastal areas largely populated by the dominant, highly educated castes, while the mountainous areas and plateaux are inhabited mainly by tribal people, many of whom live below the poverty line (Gupta 2002; Mishra 2010). The SC and ST groups constitute 41% of the total population of the state. While Orissa's infant mortality rate is comparable with that of Rajasthan (69/1000 live births), its maternal mortality ratio (303/100,000) is somewhat better (Sample Registration System (SRS) 2004–2006). Malaria remains the major cause of child deaths in Orissa (Gupta 2002). Gender relations among the tribal peoples are more equitable than in the Hindu caste society. The study district in south Orissa is home to more than 62 distinctive indigenous groups who form almost 50% of its population. The ST groups are internally relatively less hierarchically organised than is the norm for Hindu caste society. People live off the land and forest, and trade has been relatively less common. The area originally inhabited by the tribal groups had a troubled relationship with the British colonial authorities, who sought to eradicate many social customs and to reform rules governing ownership and use of land and forest (see Pathy 1995; Mishra 2010). The post-colonial Indian government carried on in the spirit of this colonial legacy, reframing it in the name of 'mainstreaming' tribal communities through a series of social welfare and development schemes. Religiously, many groups still adhere to local forms of animism and ancestral worship, although conversions to Hinduism and Christianity have occurred in some places.

The three rounds of the district level Household and Facility Survey (conducted by the Ministry of Health and Welfare, and collecting district-level information on reproductive and maternal health, family planning, child health, and health service utilisation) show that immunisation coverage in both Orissa and Rajasthan has been consistently increasing over the past 5 years (DLHS-3, 2007–2008). Based on the DLHS-3 report, full immunisation coverage in Orissa increased from 53.5% in 2000–1 to 62.4% in 2007–8, BCG coverage from 90.4% to 94.2%, and measles coverage from 67.9% to 81.1%. However, the percentage of those fully immunised among the tribal population (44.5%) is much lower than for the state as a whole.

While India is a subcontinent of federative states, with a huge, more or less homogeneous health system, Malawi is smaller than either Rajasthan or Orissa in terms both of area and population. It is a subSaharan, landlocked African country with an area of 118,484 km^2 (including Lake Malawi). The country has a population of 13.9 million people with 2.8% annual population growth (Malawi National Statistical Office 2011). The infant mortality rate was 73 per thousand live births in 2010; an improvement from 134 in 1992 (Malawi National Statistical Office 2011). Malawi is therefore on course to meet MDG4 of reducing infant mortality by 2015. Such progress is attributed, among others factors, to access to immunisation and increased use of insecticide-treated bed nets (UNDP 2011). Serious challenges, however, remain. In 2011 UNDP ranked Malawi 171st out of 181 countries on the human development index. The life expectancy is only 54.2 years, while 12% people aged 15–49 years are living with HIV (UNDP 2011). The country has a high prevalence of malnutrition: 41% stunting rate, 17% underweight, and 64% of children aged 6–59 months are anaemic. The maternal mortality ratio of 807 per 100,000 is among the highest in Africa. Human resources for health are desperately lacking, with a 74% vacancy rate for nurses in 2010 (World Health Organization 2011a) and a 62% vacancy rate for doctors (2007). There are only two physicians and 38 nurses per 100, 000 population (WHO 2011). Access to health services is limited: only 46% of the population lives within 5 km of a health facility (WHO 2009). About 60% of total health expenditure comes from external sources, 2.7% from private insurance, and 9% is out-of-pocket expenditure (World Health Organization 2009c). It is estimated that 90% of the population has no access to electricity, with the percentage rising to 95% in rural areas (World Bank 2010).

Despite its many challenges, the country's commitment to immunisation and its impressive immunisation coverage have often been noted as a success story. Since Malawi attained the UCI goal in 1989, immunisation coverage for all target diseases has been said to be maintained at 80% or more. A recent league table prepared by UNICEF finds Malawi ranking 16th out of 53 African states for its 84% coverage of the third dose of DTP3 vaccine in children (Bowie et al. 2006).

The country is divided into three regions, containing 28 districts and 22 district hospitals. There are four central hospitals which act as the top most referral hospitals. Furthermore, there are 414 public primary healthcare facilities and

138 non-profit and for-profit health facilities, with a majority of the latter belonging to CHAM (Richardson et al. 2009).

Fieldwork was conducted in the two districts of Dowa and Thyolo. Dowa district is located in the central region of Malawi, some 53 km from Lilong-we, the capital city. It has an area of 3041 km^2 and a population of 573, 935 (Malawi National Statistical Office 2011). With its population of 132,005 women of child-bearing age (15–45), the district expects 28,697 deliveries per year. There are 28,697 children under the age of 1 (Malawi National Statistical Office 2011). Dowa district has 212 immunisation sites, of which 28 are static. Of these, 21 belong to the MoH, four to CHAM, one to the United Nations High Commissioner for Refugees (UNHCR, which runs a refugee camp in the area), one to an NGO, whilst one is run privately. The district has 184 outreach clinics, with the MoH owning 144 of them. CHAM has 26 sites, UNHCR has five, four are run privately, while five are run by NGOs (MoH 2010). According to the Malawi National Statistical Office (2011), 82.7% of children in the district received all basic vaccinations: BCG, measles and three doses each of DPT or pentavalent DPT-HepB-Hib and polio vaccine (excluding polio given at birth). The infant mortality rate is 64% compared to the national rate of 73%, while the female literacy rate of 64.2% is slightly lower than the national rate of 67.6% (Malawi National Statistical Office 2011).

Dowa district is predominantly populated by Chewa people, followed by a Ngoni minority. The Yao are mainly found in trading centres within the district. Dowa is an agricultural district growing cash crops such as tobacco, cotton, and groundnuts. Food crops include maize (the major food crop), sweet potatoes, and pulses. The Chewa are matrilineal, while the Ngonis have a patrilineal kinship system. In this district we conducted interviews at three MoH facilities, including the district hospital. We also undertook fieldwork in two villages. At the health facilities we talked to medical doctors, clinicians, nurses, HSAs, medical assistants, and health management information system (HMIS) officers. In one of the villages we talked to chiefs, grandmothers, mothers and caretakers, and men including husbands and traditional birth attendants. In another village, where one member of our research team stayed with a family, we conducted fieldwork for 6 months. We also joined supervisors and observed Child Health Week activities across the district.

Thyolo district in the Southern region has an area of 1715 km^2 and a population of 617,195. According to the district HMIS officer, there are 27 health facilities that report to his office based at the district hospital. Eighteen of these belong to the MoH, with CHAM having nine facilities. There are also 17 health facilities belonging to tea and macadamia plantations, while five health facilities are run privately. The 17 facilities belonging to plantations do not report to the district hospital, but to the nearest health facility belonging to either the MoH or CHAM.

The Malawi National Statistical Office (2011) reports that 86.7% of children in Thyolo district received all basic vaccinations. The infant mortality rate is 77, slightly higher than the national rate. Tea estates cover a large part of the district, occupying a lot of cultivable land. As such, many people earn their livelihood through tea plucking. Land is so scarce that some people are being relocated to other districts. The district is populated by several tribes, including the Ngoni, Yao, and Lhomwe, with the last-named being in the majority. As in Dowa, there is a mixture of matrilineal and patrilineal kinship systems, with a dominance of matrilineality. In Thyolo we conducted fieldwork at four health facilities, including the district hospital, several outreaches, and three villages. Two of our research team members conducted fieldwork for 6 months. They were hosted by nurses with whom they stayed, and they followed HSAs to outreach clinics. One of the members conducted interviews at the district hospital, at a health centre, and in a village, while two members had brief visits to the district hospital and the communities. In the course of our fieldwork we observed several outreach clinics, talked to medical doctors, clinicians, nurses, HSAs, HMIS officers, chiefs, grandmothers, mothers and caretakers, husbands and traditional birth attendants.

In both Dowa and Thyolo, chiefs are prominent figures. There is a hierarchy of chiefs in all districts of Malawi. At the top stands the paramount chief, who rules over an entire tribe or ethnic group. In some cases such paramount chiefs are based in other countries or districts but their jurisdiction is still recognised by their subjects. For instance, the paramount chief for the Chewa of Malawi, Mozambique, and Zambia is based in Zambia. Several ranks follow, from the paramount chief to the lowest traditional leader, who looks after a single village. Chiefs in Malawi are on the government payroll, and thus represent both tradition and the state. They are, however, under pressure to toe the line of the ruling political party. Chiefs are central in mobilising their communities for local development, including immunisation, and their role can become crucial, as it did during the 2010 measles outbreak that we discussed in Chapter 5.

Our three study sites in India and Malawi thus differ from one another in numerous respects. An examination of their 'vaccination cultures' will help us understand both how immunisation practices are influenced by these distinctive local contexts, and also 'what lies behind the numbers'. Why, in other words, does Malawi achieve consistently high immunisation coverage whilst India displays such variation between states, districts, and ethnic communities?

Policy contexts: the materiality of state practices

Although immunisation largely follows a global agenda, as we have argued throughout this book, in the local community it appears as a state intervention: one among many. The national–local interface is where we can begin to understand how the state makes itself routinely visible through its material practices, the ideas it promulgates and the people who represent it, and how such visibility affects immunisation delivery and outcome.

We will show how through its routine bureaucratic practices (including the recruitment of village-level health workers, health passports or immunisation cards, cash incentives, welfare schemes, and the distribution of medicines) the verticality of the state ('up there', 'above society') is made 'effective and authoritative' (Ferguson and Gupta 2002, p. 983). For the local community, engaging with vaccine entails an engagement with the state. It entails citizenship.

In India, legitimate allegiance to the state situates vaccine and vaccination in a moral and political discourse—as the right thing for a modern and rational citizen to do. Nevertheless, and despite the similarity of vaccination practices, local communities perceive the state in quite different ways: the result of historical contingencies, of perceived vulnerabilities, and of social relations within the community. Images of a benevolent state, common among the tribal communities of Orissa, contrast with those of a modern yet potentially untrustworthy state found among many Muslim and Hindu groups in Rajasthan.

The routine, bureaucratic practices of the state are legitimised through national policies, said to articulate the interests of the 'nation'. So far as contemporary Indian immunisation practices are concerned, one needs to take into account the recent policy shift under the NRHM (NRHM 2005–2012). The EPI was introduced to India in 1978. It focused mainly on urban areas until 1985, when the programme was extended nationwide and renamed the UIP. As part of large-scale health sector reforms NRHM was launched in 2005 in order to undertake 'architectural correction' of the state public health system in rural areas. It aims to provide affordable, equitable, and accessible health care to women and children living in rural areas. One of the goals of NRHM is to reduce infant and maternal mortality rates in line with India's commitment to MDG4 and MDG5.

The recent policy of NRHM has three significant implications for the way in which immunisation services are delivered. First, it regularises immunisation practices (a fixed day of the month in a village). Second, it involves recruitment of a new cadre of lay health workers (the ASHAs) from among village women. They are offered cash incentives for motivating the community to access and utilise healthcare services (immunisation, antenatal care, institutional delivery). Third, NRHM includes stricter monitoring of all components of the health services falling under the Mission. The key mechanism now promoted by the state to ensure better coverage is the village immunisation day. Through focusing on the immunisation day we can best unravel the dynamics through which coverage data are produced, and we can explore how vaccination behaviour relates to the larger sociopolitical context of state–citizen relationships.

Policy in Malawi has evolved somewhat differently. EPI was initiated in Malawi in 1976 as a pilot programme and became fully operational in 1978 (MoH 2003). Only smallpox vaccine was given on a large scale before 1973, while DPT and BCG vaccinations were provided in a few health centres (Chilowa and Munthali 1998). Differently from India, EPI has always had a strong rural focus in Malawi. The fact that it secured a degree of independence as a vertical programme within the MoH has been identified as key to its success (Eie 2008, p. 44). While UNICEF is responsible for procurement of vaccines on the government's behalf, EPI has primary responsibility for their distribution, as well as for routine vaccination practices carried out by HSAs.

Since January 2002, when pentavalent vaccine (DPT-HepB-Hib) was introduced in Malawi, the EPI has offered measles, DPT-HepB-Hib, polio and BCG vaccines to children under 1 year, and tetanus toxoid to women who are either pregnant or of child-bearing age. Vitamin A supplementation is administered alongside immunisation services (Malawi Ministry of Health 2003). In November 2011 the programme introduced pneumococcal conjugate vaccine, which fitted into the existing vaccination schedule. As in India, immunisation activities are carried out along with other services, which include growth monitoring, family planning, nutrition, health education, and early treatment of ailments at the under-5 clinics (MoH 2002).

Since 2004, when Malawi adopted the SWAp, the EPI has been considered one of the central programmes for delivery of the EHP within the SWAp (Hutton and Tanner 2004; MoH 2004a). Malawi's EHP focuses on the major causes of disease and death in the country: vaccine-preventable diseases, malaria, maternal and neonatal morbidity and mortality, tuberculosis, acute respiratory infections, acute diarrheal diseases, sexually transmitted infections, schistosomiasis, nutritional deficiencies, eye, ear and skin infections, and common injuries (MoH 2004b). Targeting these diseases is considered to be in the interests of poor people, and the EHP is viewed as an instrument of poverty alleviation as articulated in the Malawi Growth and Development Strategy. This in turn is linked to the MDGs, and the EPI is viewed as key to the delivery of MDG4.

Despite the major differences between the health delivery systems in India and Malawi, health workers play a key role in each country's vaccine delivery rituals. However, as we will see, system differences influence the way in which they work.

Delivering vaccines: rituals of routine immunisation days and outreach vaccination clinics

A routine immunisation day in Orissa (India)

In a small relatively homogenous tribal village in Orissa on the third Wednesday of the month the ASHA is busy visiting houses to remind parents to bring their children to the immunisation site. It is early morning, women villagers are busy going to the river to collect water, and some are trying to finish cooking before going to work in their fields, or for some to the nearby mines. The ASHA and the AWW are waiting for the ANM to arrive. The ANM arrives after collecting the vaccines from the PHC. She travels on a motorbike, accompanied by her husband. She takes out a rough sheet of paper which lists the names of children against the recommended vaccines. The health workers gather at a public space (pre-school crèche, school premises, veranda of the AWW helper) in the village. The ASHA worker herself, or the neighbours or relatives (whoever is available) bring the children to the immunisation site. It is peak agricultural season, so some mothers have already left for the fields by the time the ANM reaches the village. This results in a 'passing the buck' game between the ASHA/AWW and ANM, each blaming the other for not doing a good job of retaining the people. Some of the mothers/kin don't bring the immunisation card. The ANM then sends someone (sometimes the grown-up children who come to watch) to run to get the card from the child's house. The ANM then vaccinates the child. She carries a huge box of iron syrup bottles, which she hands over to the ASHA for distribution to pregnant women. She also hands over medicines like choloroquine. One woman has come to the ANM complaining of fever and is given some medicines. Another comes complaining of night blindness. In such a manner, people come and go with different concerns and at different times. Meanwhile the ASHA has told the ANM that Mrs X refuses to bring her grandchild for vaccination. Like the rest of her family she believes that the child would get fever on being vaccinated, and this would disrupt the household and agricultural work. The ASHA is told to talk to the child's mother (who earlier had gone to the river for water) instead. The mother says that she has no idea what her mother-in-law had said. The ASHA persuades the mother to come to the ANM and explain. The ANM assures the mother that she'll give paracetamol to reduce fever and there is nothing to worry about. She then vaccinates the child and gives paracetamol. As the vaccination session unfolds some people come and go, some

---

A routine immunisation day in Orissa (India) *(continued)*

stay behind to chat, others come in a hurry and ask to be treated quickly, pushing their child into the arms of one of the health workers.

After the vaccination session is over, it is time to update the records. The ANM makes ticks on a piece of paper on which she had written the names of children to be vaccinated. She later finalises the list, which is submitted every month to the PHC. The AWW copies the record from her, explaining to the researcher that 'both sets of records have to be same, otherwise we will be in trouble, the medical record at the health centres and the records of the Department of Child and Women Development are checked and tallied later in a common platform; if anything goes wrong, we will be questioned'. The AWW and ASHA also discuss any malnourished child that needs treatment and get the form signed by the ANM for referral.

In Rajasthan, the session proceeded very similarly. What were officially called MCHN days—or what the patients called simply 'vaccination' (tika karan)—were held at the angan wadi centres (village child-care centres). Here, on the same day, the AWW would weigh children and distribute nutritious supplements to lactating mothers and families with small children.

An outreach vaccination clinic in Thyolo district (Malawi)

After a rainy night the HSAs start to push their bicycles through the muddy paths on their way to a vaccination day at a village health centre. A small coolbox with icepacks, vaccine vials, diluents, mixing syringes, auto-destructible syringes, and a hanging scale and registers is strapped to the back of the bikes, together with a cardboard safety box for used syringes. After a long climb up steep, muddy, mountain paths they reach the village. There's already a long queue outside the nursery. The pink health passports are laid out in a long row on the ground, indicating the owner's place in the queue. The local village health committee, a non-salaried local group, or person greets them. When the equipment is unpacked there's a sigh of relief when the vaccines are brought out. Often there are limited or no vaccines to bring and the mothers will leave in disappointment. A few people run off to inform others that the vaccines have arrived this time. Immediately after arrival, the scale is set up and the weighing of children and recording of their weights in the health

An outreach vaccination clinic in Thyolo district (Malawi) *(continued)*

passports starts. The passports are then taken to another table where the numbers are copied into a register. Two HSAs sit at a bench with the health passports trying to figure out which vaccines each child should receive. As the line in front of the scale shrinks an HSA stands up, claps his hands, and starts singing a chorus that includes instructions on family planning and the blessings of vaccinations. The mothers and children who had scattered all over the area quickly return once the singing starts. Three songs are sung before someone suggests a prayer. The senior HSA then embarks on a spirited 'health talk' on responsible parenthood, the need for continued growth monitoring and vaccinations after 12 months; the latter was a challenge for the health workers. As he speaks he continuously moves about in the crowd, sometimes capturing the mothers' attention by scolding them for inappropriate behaviour. He also talks about the measles epidemic affecting the area at the time. He asks individuals in the crowd to name symptoms and preventive actions to take, while repeating the correct answers and encouraging those present to spread the information, 'reminding each other of what we know'. The information on preventive practices includes references to the blessings of herbal remedies and 'raising the mat' (see below), a traditional practice of sexual abstention, which the HSA endorses since the outreach was conducted in the midst of a measles epidemic. A murmur of disappointment arises when he ends by explaining that there would be no measles vaccination that day, since they had not received any vaccines. After the health talk it is time for vaccination. The mothers with children are called up one by one according to the order of the health passports. The mothers called forward sit down on a bench, turn over the pink health passport, and uncover the thigh of the children. Once a BCG injection is called for and a junior HSA calls for a more experienced colleague to set the needle. While the procedures are unfolding, some children are breastfed to stop them crying, while others crawl around. People come and go continuously. They discuss local events and they talk about their worries over the fevers and swellings their children experienced after the last round of vaccinations. One mother is scolded for not bringing the health passports, another one for skipping the previous round of vaccinations. A third mother has forgotten her own health passport and is given a shot of tetanus toxoid. Her scared face is met with laughter and friendly teasing from the crowd. After a few hours the session comes to an end. The ground is filled with syringe wrapping paper and with small puddles where the children have urinated. (Adapted from Alfsen 2011, with permission of the author.)

These excerpts from our observations in each country indicate the central role played by health workers in both. The Indian setting, however, involves three categories of health worker, making for a more complex dynamic, both between the health workers and the local community and among the health workers themselves. For example, as the excerpts suggest, mutual blaming is common when planned activities fail (villagers not showing up for immunisation, for example). After all, ASHAs are recruited specifically in order to mobilise the community to access public health services (and according to the official narrative, immunisation coverage has indeed increased as a result).

The disorder of the immunisation day in India contrasts with Malawi's relatively disciplined and organised outreach clinic. The clinic becomes a collective ritual evoking morality through prayers and health songs. The morality invoked (and evoked) around immunisation meshes with the more general moral order: belief in God, the desirability of striving for a public good, and the traditional practice of 'raising the mat'. (Metaphorically, the everyday act of rolling up the straw sleeping mat and raising it up against the wall implies abstaining from sex in the household. This is done to prevent transmission of misfortunes from parents to child, which might occur when sexually active people touch infants. Symptoms of swelling fever, ill health in general or at times following vaccination are believed to be the result of contact with a sexually active person). Legitimacy for vaccination is sought from other sources that are traditionally convincing and/or compelling. Singing health songs is a long-standing practice in most parts of Africa. The HSAs use them to evoke a sense of 'community' (with repeated reference to 'we') and the collective well-being. Although the HSAs direct the singing they take care to include the audience, leaving much of the initiative in their hands, pulling them into collective processes promoting vaccination and general health information as a public good in the process. Immunisation in India, on the other hand, is part of the routine and mundane activities of the village. As we saw in the excerpts, ASHAs might be running around reminding parents. Where the mother has left for the fields, a grandmother, young paternal aunt or another female relative would often be the one who brings the child for vaccination. Health or vaccination talk, e.g. discussions about symptoms of diseases or supply of vaccines, common in the outreach clinic in Malawi, is conspicuous by its absence in the Indian context. Thus whilst vaccination remains the focus of collective attention in the Malawi site, this focus is far more diffuse in the sites we observed in India.

The health passport in Malawi and the immunisation card in India (also known as the mother–child health card) serve the same broad purpose. Through recording health information and promoting adherence to national health programmes both enable state surveillance—the 'practices through which states reproduce spatial orders and scalar hierarchies' (Ferguson and Gupta 2002, p. 984). However the ways in which they are used differ.

In Malawi the health passport is seen, and literally spoken of, as a 'ticket' to receiving proper health services for children (Seljeskog et al. 2006). As the excerpts above indicate, the passports establish the legitimacy of Malawi mothers as state subjects, and hence as legitimate beneficiaries of state services. Without the proof of vaccination evidenced in the health passport, the child may not be allowed to receive other health services. These passports function as part of the queue system at the under-5 clinics. When people arrive in the morning, many having walked long distances with a child on their back, they put their health passport in a pile or line indicating the order of arrival. In the woman's passport there are drawings and short texts on how a man should take care of his family, and information on proper tuberculosis treatment. While the child's health passport contains information in the tribal languages on breastfeeding, the adult's passport contains information on HIV testing and treatment. The care taken to wrap the vaccination cards in paper or plastic wrappers underlines the value attached to them. If the health passport is left behind there could be negative repercussions for the mother. Most mothers do not dare to present their children for treatment if their health passports do not show proof of vaccination. Health passports thus become a means to assert biological citizenship for the Malawi community.

The immunisation cards in India do not seem to be treated with quite the same respect, nor are they linked to receipt of other health services (except the promotion of institutional delivery through cash incentives available both to mothers-to-be and ASHAs). Under the NRHM the immunisation card was renamed the mother and child safety card, and now contains information on the antenatal care of women, post-partum care, immunisation schedule, and information on child care, including breast feeding. We observed during the immunisation days in both Indian states that sometimes immunisation cards are kept by the ANMs to ensure that her records are in place. In fact in the majority of the cases, the ANMs keep a spare record of names of eligible mothers and children for vaccination lest the parents lose the cards. Like the parents, the health workers themselves are also under state surveillance. While some do bring the card to the immunisation site, many mothers forget it, with the result that the ANM or ASHA sends a child to fetch it. Many women did not have any special place to keep these cards safely. In some houses they were kept in grainbaskets. Other women had them under their mattress or in the suitcase where their clothes were also kept. Recently in Orissa the card has been linked to support for the education of a girl child. If the girl child has been fully immunised she becomes eligible for 100,000 rupees (US$1806) towards her education. The cards need to be produced as proof. We observed that parents/caretakers treat the card as an entrance ticket to access these material benefits and keep them till they receive the money. ASHAs and AWWs periodically remind them of this: 'Keep the card. If you don't show it in the hospital, you will not receive the money.'

Vaccines as part of a larger package of health services: process of cumulative trust

Vaccines reach the community through a larger health package that typically includes the promotion of antenatal services, institutional delivery, and family planning services. This has two implications. First, through offering a range of services the state makes itself much more visible. Potentially at least, a moral image of the state as benefactor and protector of its citizens is created. Compliance, displaying good citizenship, then seems more appropriate. Such government strategies are good examples of what the anthropologist Aihwa Ong (2007) calls 'technologies of subjection': techniques that are used to change population behaviour through laws, incentives, and disincentives that will influence a person's choices rather than trying to change attitudes or knowledge directly. Second, this 'packaging' makes it easier for health workers to motivate the community. The material benefits attaching to some services (for example the cash payments Indian families receive for institutional delivery) are used by health workers in the Indian context to generate compliance to vaccination and overall trust in their services.

In Malawi too offering a range of services means that some services can be used to stimulate use of others. Our research suggests, however, that this works differently in the two contexts. In Malawi it seems that other services ride on the back of vaccination, in direct contrast to the situation in India. We see this, for example, when health workers struggle to keep mothers coming to the under-5 clinics after the measles vaccine has been administered at 9 months. Besides vaccination, family planning services also act as an incentive in Malawi. For instance, clinics that include family planning in their services are more attractive and well utilised. Providing a range of services all at once also serves Malawi well considering the country's acute shortage of health workers (cf. Nyirenda and Flikke, 2012). In India, on the contrary, curative services act as hooks for vaccination—and sometimes for discussing family planning—creating demand for and trust in health workers' services or through creation of social bonds and reciprocity obligations. Providing a range of services is a means of achieving visibility. It should not be seen as merely a way of compensating for shortages in health personnel.

Distribution of medicines for the treatment of minor ailments is an important and visible part of the larger health service package. There is a huge demand for curative medicines in both the Indian and the Malawian communities, and villagers can often be seen asking health workers to give them medicines against fever, diarrhoea, and skin diseases. This demand is often encouraged by the health workers, especially when they are expected to distribute medicines as part of a government programme of disease control. For example in Orissa, tuberculosis, malaria, diarrhoea, pneumonia, and leprosy are diseases which all require urgent attention. (In Malawi this is also true of HIV/AIDS.) Distribution of medicines bestows authority on health workers, allowing them to sustain their role. Inadequate supply of medicines is therefore a major concern voiced by many ASHAs at their monthly meetings. In Orissa, we observed that vaccine response is much better in villages where health workers have successfully established such a culture of medicine by distributing medicines door-to-door or by ensuring an adequate supply. Conversely, the ANM's role is often criticised by villagers, saying she shows up only on immunisation day and does not offer curative services. Through satisfying the demand for curative services (i.e. treatment of diseases) willingness to accept preventive measures is enhanced. While HSAs in Malawi give medicines for other ailments, such as uncomplicated malaria, the demand for vaccines is not linked to such services. Nevertheless, the ability to provide such medicines enhances the HSAs' reputation.

In India, we observed that health workers often went further still, offering other kinds of services in order to elicit and sustain trust in the community. For example, in Orissa the ASHA workers offered information on all other government programmes, and they cooperated and actively participated in traditional rituals organised by individual households. In a similar vein, one particularly successful motivator in Rajasthan was actively helping and assisting anyone who needed to go to hospital or to certain healers, for whatever reason. Another would help her fellow villagers with reading or with filling in government forms or responding to official letters. Community members refer to a health worker as 'sister', and trust in the health worker may translate into trust in the services she provides. Social obligations are thus important: many women say 'we get our children immunised as ASHA sister has said this'. However, such acts of reciprocity cannot be taken for granted but need to be cautiously and carefully nurtured by active and creative ASHAs and ANMs.

However, trust is not elicited through offering services alone. The offering of services is itself enmeshed in social relations, and in India such relations may be marked by differentiation along caste, ethnicity, gender, and class lines. In Rajasthan villages are characterised by such differences, and the ASHA's ability to perform her tasks is contingent on her and her family's relationship to other villagers, her caste, and her class status. At some houses she is welcomed and has time to explain her errand. Other houses she does not enter and messages have to be exchanged. In yet other houses a passing child is used to convey a message to the inhabitants. Personal and family histories, and histories of social relations in the community, provide the lens through which people (including the ASHAs) interpret information and events (such as the appearance of the ANM in the village on a non-vaccination day or a complaining client). An ANM residing in a local town would have to spend more energy attaining such close relations and trust in the local population and a lot would depend on her willingness and ability to do so.

In Malawi, an HSA's knowledge of the local context is also crucial, both for his or her capacity to relay health messages in an appropriate manner, and for his or her acceptance in the local community. Although HSAs are regarded as representing the formal health system, their regular interaction with community members and participation in local community activities, such as church services and funerals, integrates them in the community. (New recruitment arrangements, whereby HSAs are not necessarily recruited from the same areas, might make their integration into local communities more difficult.) We see something similar in tribal Orissa. Where ASHAs are themselves members of the tribal community, actively participating in community rituals such as traditional child protection rituals, this gives added legitimacy to their role as state agents. The two sets of expectations can also come into conflict. A tribal community may expect the ASHA or AWW to actively participate in and support a traditional ritual that is actively discouraged by the state. As a state employee the ASHA, a 'social health activist', should be promoting modern medicine at the expense of what may be viewed officially as quackery. While for the state, traditional and modern stand as dichotomous and in opposition to one another, for a tribal community in Orissa vaccination may appear wholly compatible with the rituals of protecting the womb and the child. In this case the tension does not have any consequence for the ASHA. In other circumstances we have seen how the ASHA's loyalty to the community, and conflicting pressure from superiors and obligations towards the state, may put her in quite a vulnerable position (Gjøstein 2012).

The package of services that the health worker is required to provide can be used to negotiate the trust of the community. But roles and commitment to health schemes other than vaccination can also have consequences beyond the control of the individual health worker (Das and Das 2003). This is particularly true of the various family planning programmes. In India, health workers experience heavy pressure from their superiors to achieve monthly targets for sterilisations and IUDs (intrauterine devices, i.e. copper T) insertions. Adverse experiences with such family planning measures often translate into distrust of the health workers, who would have painstakingly convinced the women to adopt the specific family planning service. This is not limited to family planning measures. Distrust of ASHA workers in tribal Orissa can often arise when they mobilise and accompany women to health centres for delivery only to find that the health centre is ill equipped to handle delivery cases and they are then referred to distant district hospitals.

Delivery of vaccination as a good or a service is thus situated in a context of other health and non-health services. Favourable responses have to be negotiated and sustained through a process of cumulatively building trust in which this whole package is implicated. This trust-building is more problematic in India than in Malawi: a consequence of the socially segmented nature of the villages studied, of historical experiences with the state and its programmes, and of the ways in which vaccine delivery is organised. Ferguson and Gupta (2002) point out the paradox of the village-level state workers. Being part of the community they find it difficult to assert the verticality of the state apparatus yet at the same time, being marginal members of the state bureaucracy, they are themselves subject to surveillance and monitoring from above. Their paradoxical situation is explicated in the following section, in which we discuss how health workers face pressures from the state to meet immunisation targets and ensure coverage.

Being a 'good and efficient' health worker: ensuring coverage

Data on immunisation coverage are used not only as a proxy for health system performance and the success or failure of public health programmes, they are also used as performance indicators for the village-level health workers (Coutinho et al. 2000; George 2009). On the basis of numbers such as children vaccinated or women registered for antenatal care or delivering in hospital, a health worker is labelled as good and efficient or as underperforming. Although there may be no immediate negative sanction for lack of performance, subtle (yet coercive) pressures are brought to bear. In India there are positive pressures: inducements such as a cash prize for a good worker, and a 'best ASHA award' for having the maximum coverage in her catchment area. Negative sanctions include public ridicule in meetings. In India, ASHAs gather with their ANMs in a monthly meeting at the sector level, led by sector medical officers (MOs). The ANMs and MOs in turn gather every month at the next administrative level (the block level), led by the block chief medical officer (BCMO). Our observations of some of these meetings showed that the village workers (the ASHAs and ANMs) were made to sit on the floor while the seniors sat on chairs or behind desks and lectured them, questioned them about calculation of targets, urged them to achieve higher numbers, and had 'high' or 'low' performers stand up to report and receive praise or scolding. Such target and reporting pressures can be observed all the way up to the top state levels, and the target-based programmes clearly dominate the whole health system.

Although health workers are responsible for a variety of tasks (an ANM is supposed to maintain 15 different registers on aspects of mother–child health and disease surveillance), performance is judged on selected key indicators. These include the number of antenatal care check-ups (indicated through two tetanus toxoid shots given to the mothers), the number of institutional deliveries, the number of sterilisation cases, attendance at immunisation days, and the number of children and pregnant mothers actually vaccinated at the sessions. The significance of these indicators is repeatedly emphasised in different forums. ANMs interpreted the recent policy of NRHM in terms of more and stricter supervision of record maintenance. One ANM remarked: 'NRHM is about producing more and more records . . . it is not the work per se but the nature of doing the work that has changed'. She expanded further:

> It is a human tendency that if one does the same work monotonously for a long time, one tends to become lax. NRHM has introduced rigour and stricter means to do the work we were doing earlier. Look at this Immunization chart. Immunization was always there. We used to talk about high and low coverage but never gave a thought to how to better that coverage. NRHM has introduced those methods of calculating the number of 'left outs' and 'drop outs' so that it becomes easier to tap when people do drop out, and where. It gives a better and clear picture about Immunization coverage. However NRHM has also brought about several other schemes, which increases the paper work and load of reports. Imagine, I have to make these extra reports. I maintain 8 different reports. NRHM makes us produce more and more records. When one has to make so many reports, it is natural that people start cheating.

Another ANM added:

> Immunization work was always there. But there was no fixed day like this, we could come whenever we had time and we could go to individual households and inject the children; but now, Immunization days are fixed and it is mandatory for us to be here. Also there was no work of paper and pen earlier. We had to write on a piece of paper and show it to our senior as evidence that we did our work. Now we have to make systematic records.

One of the ASHA health workers spoke of the qualities required of a good health worker:

> An ASHA should have the ability to co-operate with others, she should be someone whom people can rely on and trust, she should have the capability of explaining things

she gets to know in the meetings, and importantly she should have the patience to take all the scolding of one's seniors when records are not updated or performance is not that good.

In Malawi, HSAs and district health workers are also under pressure to meet targets. Most regard the recording and reporting of coverage data as extra work. This perception is amplified by the fact that the HSAs, who consist of the bulk of health workers at health facilities, are also required to record data and report for other disease or health programmes. Thus, they are supposed to report to the Tuberculosis Control Programme, to the Malaria Control Programme, and to the HIV/AIDS Programme, among others. The different disease programmes each have coordinators at the district hospital and each coordinator relies on the same HSAs to provide reports. Besides reporting to the different disease and health programmes, the health facilities are also required to compile reports for the HMIS office at the district hospital. In some instances, such reporting pressure leads the HSAs and other health workers to resort to deliberate manipulation of data.

As explained by one health manager:

> Some health centres cook up data. During reporting, they see the trend and make conclusions without focusing on all the data. For instance, if they see 6 malaria cases on page 1, five cases on page 2 and four cases on page 3 they come up with the average and conclude on the number of cases from 10 pages.

In Malawi, the pressure and struggle regarding numbers surfaced in a revealing manner during an MSF-led vaccination campaign in the midst of the measles epidemic in 2010 (Ommundsen 2011).

Capturing and reporting the 'truth': the struggle for numbers during epidemics

In May 2010 MSF started a vaccination campaign in Malawi in order to quench the full-blown epidemic that was spreading through Southern Africa. The Malawian Department of Health had insisted that the international units from MSF used the local HSAs in the campaign. The MSF field supervisor in this case was a European nurse. Ideally the HSAs should live in the communities they were responsible for, and thus have a very good overview of the demography and general health in their catchment area. At this particular instance they established vaccination sites at local churches and schools, and vaccinated all children between the ages of 6 months and 15 years of age—regardless of previous vaccination status. The campaign was carried out together with an

Capturing and reporting the 'truth': the struggle for numbers during epidemics *(continued)*

annual vitamin-A and abendazole campaign. A lot of friction had occurred over payments, since the regular remuneration for the annual campaign was 800 kw (Malawian kwacha) (US$5.25 in 2010), yet the payment for the campaign was 500 kw, making the extra work lead to a factual loss of income. The HSAs had worked hard spreading information in their catchment areas about the campaign and when and where to meet. The actual turnout was way below the expectations of the MSF, who were working from the Malawian MoH's census data. Although the local HSAs emphatically stated the official numbers were wrong, and our researchers confirmed that all the targeted areas were covered, extra outreach teams were mobilised to go out and check and vaccinate all unvaccinated children they came across. One team came back at the end of the day, not having found a single unvaccinated. The other team returned having vaccinated more than a hundred children. The fatigued MSF leader praised the latter team. Incidentally the team that did not vaccinate any children was the one joined by our researcher. Once MSF had left the area it became obvious that the 'successful team' had vaccinated adults outside the target group in order to please MSF and 'get them off their back'.

In addition uncertain numbers produced at the vaccination sites marred this campaign. The local HSAs were working under pressure, continuously being under supervision and, according to our observations, harassed by the European MSF representative in front of their own people, for their lack of skill and knowledge. This created a hostile atmosphere with a lot of distrust and stress regarding expectations of output. In one case the MSF representative, sensibly enough, wanted to gather the vials at the end of the day in order to count them and measure them against the tally sheets, and prevent them being sold and used to sell fake vaccinations on the black market. The vials, however, had already been sold to bike-repair men who used them to store glue—a fact that was not revealed to the MSF representative out of fear of being fired. In addition, we know that the tally sheets on a regular basis were being adjusted in order to keep a proper balance between the two. One day an informal look at the tally sheets showed more than 700 children vaccinated, yet the vials indicated about 500. (Adapted from Ommundsen 2011, with permission of the author.)

Even though the measles campaign was an extraordinary event, it illustrates the practical problems that run through day-to-day vaccine delivery in Malawi. The expectations of numbers put on the workers at different levels, with the ensuing mistrust, creating an atmosphere in which workers did what they had to do to keep their jobs, while performing according to their own knowledge or expectations. This campaign accentuates how immunisation programmes succumb to vertical pressures rather than responding to the actual targeted children.

Often the pressure for performance encourages the health worker to shift blame onto the community. Both in Rajasthan and Orissa, for instance, health workers referred to those who do not get motivated easily as 'backward', 'not educated', 'useless', and 'dirty', hence subscribing to public health models in which failure to adopt a public health technology such as vaccination is attributed to general ignorance (Leach and Fairhead 2005). Rewards are given not to the health workers who communicate most effectively with people, or to those who help villagers understand the technology, but to those who can produce the highest numbers. In order to achieve targets, the ASHA or ANM may be willing to stretch the limits of what is ethically acceptable. A variety of strategies are used to push numbers up. One of the ASHA workers in a Rajasthan village explained the strategies she used to coerce people to come to the immunisation site:

> I always get them here by using different tactics. Today I told them that many kids were dying in Jaipur [capital of Rajasthan] because of diseases now. (Gjostein 2012, p. 48)

At that occasion this ASHA had told a family that eight children in Jaipur had been paralysed by polio in the preceding days. The additional strategy was to keep sitting there, refusing to leave and (subtly) insisting they should come until they agreed (Gjostein 2012).

But such tactics risk the loss of hard-won trust. The social processes through which numbers are produced point to the limitations of using 'coverage' to represent community demand. But what then is 'community demand', and how is it produced?

Response to and demand for vaccines: situating 'community demand'

The anthropologist Mark Nichter (1995) distinguishes between 'active community demand' and 'passive acceptance', arguing that in the absence of active community demand high coverage may not be sustainable. Active community demand, he explains, 'entails adherence to vaccination programs by an informed public which perceives the benefits of and need for specific vaccinations'. By contrast, 'passive acceptance denotes compliance which yields to the recommendations and social pressure' (Nichter 1995, p. 617). Nichter and others have pointed to the variety of contextual features that influence community demand. It depends, for example, on the way vaccination meshes with existing knowledge, aetiologies, and perceptions of diseases in the community, on perceived vulnerability to serious illness, on interactions with health workers, and on general perceptions of the state and the services it provides (Nichter 1995; Greenough 1995; Streefland 1995; Leach and Fairhead 2005). In the following section we attempt to unpack some of these determinants of 'demand' for vaccination and its implication for immunisation coverage.

Vaccination demand within local notions of child protection and remedies

Demand for vaccination in a community is dependent on how it fits with traditional medical knowledge systems, and with prevailing notions of disease prevention and child protection. Where infant mortality rates are high protecting its children may become a major concern for the community. For instance, the tribal community in Orissa has a history of infant and child deaths and a continuing high incidence of stillbirths. There is also a high incidence of morbidity due to malaria, diarrhoea, and fits. As a consequence child survival is a critical concern in the community, and a medical intervention such as immunisation tends to be interpreted in terms of its potential to address such concerns. Thus an analysis of responses on the reasons for vaccination in this community shows that whilst 21% (N = 43) express ignorance about what vaccine does to the child's body, the majority of respondents (61%) feel that vaccination is good for the overall health of the child. They believe that it will protect him or her from all kinds of diseases: diarrhoea, malaria, skin diseases, fits, and pains in the stomach and head. This reinforces the findings of earlier studies (Nichter 1990, 1995). Vaccination to a large extent is seen as offering protection against the common illnesses which the community experiences. Some of these, needless to say, are a result of chronic malnutrition or polluted water supplies. It is important to note here that the health workers like the ASHA sell the idea of vaccine to the community in these very terms, saying 'Why don't you come for the injections, it will help your child to get rid of fever and fits, and the health of your child will be good.' 'Immunization is good as it will protect from dangerous diseases.'

In Orissa, demand for vaccination needs to be read in the context of the organisation of social life, and most notably in relation to the world of ancestors known as duma: potentially dangerous forces that need to be periodically appeased. Almost all aspects of the life course, including pregnancy, childbirth, and diagnosis of human and animal illnesses, are linked to duma. The notion of prevention of diseases in tribal Orissa is ambiguous and responses to vaccination were described in terms that correspond better to a notion of protection. (Here we draw on Nichter's distinction between prevention and protection, where the latter is 'relative, time bound and contingent upon factors over which humans have some, but not total control' (Nichter 1995, p. 623).) Our data from the tribal community in Orissa show that although vaccination does not openly conform to the indigenous ancestral spirit (duma) theory, it is certainly talked about in terms of protecting from those illnesses which are said to be caused by duma. Community members emphasise that there are two kinds of illnesses: ordinary fever, or diarrhoea due to seasonal change, and serious illnesses, believed to be caused by superior evil forces. While the former should and can be treated through bio-medicines, the latter can only be treated by ritual specialists. The hierarchy between these different kinds of illnesses caused by different forces is expressed and reinforced in all rituals (Otten 2000, 2010; Mishra and Sarma 2011). Even the local healer—a female shaman—categorically says that diagnosis of an illness is very important. Ordinary fevers, pain, and headaches can be best treated by biomedicines. But these will fail when the illness is due to evil forces or faulty planetary positions. Such a hierarchy of illnesses is reflected in the community's sense of the efficacy and significance of ritual thread (a traditional means of protecting a child in Orissa) against that of vaccine. The purposes of these two protective measures are seen as quite different. The former is critical for child survival, enabling the child to be exposed to potentially dangerous spaces without being harmed. The latter contributes to overall child health and wellbeing. Furthermore, the former is a typical tribal custom that is mandatory, administered by a ritual specialist, and is 'ours' (desias), while the latter is administered by an ANM and is a government intervention. Thirdly, the ritual thread has more power and effectiveness; the high vulnerability of the child in its first year (in which the child is made to wear the ritual thread) legitimates the public health focus on controlling infant mortality and targeting six doses of vaccine within 1 year.

The implication of this hierarchy is that while vaccination is considered to be good, there would be resistance or avoidance if it disrupted normal activities. As shown in our brief description of the immunisation event, the resistance was precisely on this ground (fever accompanying vaccination would disrupt household and agricultural work). It is also for this reason that health workers understand that appearance at a vaccination session is related to the seasons, being notably lower during peak agricultural seasons. Due to the severe poverty in the areas covered by our study, this is to be expected; starvation is a more immediate concern than possible future diseases. But this is a very important problem, since children who do not receive vaccine boosters within the right period will not be properly immunised, and for the state vaccine coverage data point to failure when all vaccines are not given.

Although Rajasthan offers a different picture, evidence from Malawi resonates with tribal Orissa, even if the underlying reasons are different. Caretakers demanded good child health and not necessarily vaccine alone. Here too local remedies are available and widely used to ensure good maternal and child health in the villages we studied. Some traditional birth attendants (TBA) and other herbalists are central to the good health of mothers and children. The ultimate protection provided to the child is the result of a complicated and delicate process involving periods of sexual abstinence, combined with periods of successful sexual intercourse between the parents. It is believed that the semen strengthens the child and gets to the child through the mother's breast. Regardless of any remedies provided, whether locally or at the hospital, no medication can replace this process of ultimate protection. It is practiced in the villages studied in both Dowa and Thyolo, and is known as *kumuyika mwana kumalo* (which literally translates into 'putting the child in a place') or *kumutenga mwana* (literally 'taking the child'). Should this activity fail, it is believed that there is no way the child can grow up, and in case of failure medication is provided to the child. As in tribal Orissa, the villagers in these districts in Malawi insisted that there are certain illnesses that can be addressed only through local remedies while others can be addressed through biomedical means. Vaccination cannot 'put a child in place' or 'take a child'. Rituals such a 'putting a child in a place' and other remedies demonstrate the ultimate trust people have in the protective efficacy of local remedies. In Malawi, allopathic medicine is associated with Christianity and enlightenment. It can be said therefore that vaccinations take place in a sociocultural context where mechanisms, including preventive ones, are in place to ensure good child health. Although mothers juggle between different remedies, including vaccines, to protect their children, it appears that there are certain remedies that cannot be substituted under any circumstances. This is significant as it puts vaccines in a certain hierarchical order in the list of techniques available for protecting children's health, though without denying their benefits. Local and biomedical disease aetiologies were not necessarily merged in Malawi but people still sought biomedical care, including vaccination, because of an overall trust in biomedicine, a sense of normality, and entertainment attached to the activities at under-5 clinics.

Vaccination is thus situated in a complex dynamic of traditional and modern systems of medicine. The process of reinterpretation of vaccine within the traditional worldviews is also significantly linked to perceived vulnerability of individual and collective bodies. In Dowa, Malawi, it became apparent that female identity was intimately tied up in a nexus of relations to children, land,

and agricultural harvest and food (Danielsen 2011). Policy changes such as family planning, or poor harvests leading to starvation and malnourishment, affected how women felt about themselves in a manner that in turn influenced their healthcare behaviour. On the whole, family planning appears to have been accepted and sought out by Malawian mothers, although often behind the backs of their husbands. But family planning easily led to a feeling of vulnerability in a country plagued by very high child mortality. Nevertheless vaccination appears to have been conceptually bundled with family planning and mortality. However, agricultural production was spoken of as in decline; fertilisers too expensive to buy, and the land growing more and more barren, 'just like the wombs of the women'. In a context like this, malnutrition ensured a continued high mortality despite very good vaccination coverage. Women of reproductive age therefore remained very vulnerable, a situation that could easily lead to a loss of confidence in vaccination if the mortality rate does not decline.

Rajasthan offers a somewhat more complex picture, both because of the existence of a number of established systems of medicine and of a differentiated community which engages with these systems differently (Knivstoen 2012). In Rajasthan, one finds a plurality of well-established medical traditions, including Ayurveda, Unani, Siddha, homeopathy, and ancestral practices, as well as allopathic ('western') medicine (cf. Stoner 1986). In addition to these medical traditions, different strands of spirit belief as well as astrology also provide explanations of illness, and their practitioners offer curative and protective measures. Villagers commonly draw on several of these traditions. Their 'popular knowledge' (a term we prefer to the more common 'traditional' or 'local' knowledge, or to the still more judgmental notion of 'beliefs') of health and illness, the knowledge villagers share and discuss, is thus highly eclectic. But this wide range of choices, advice, and experts creates uncertainty among parents and grandparents as they seek to ensure their own or their children's health. Experience may have taught them that they should not always turn to allopathic medicine. Their trust in that particular medical system may have been eroded by experience of the poor quality of government health services or lack of access. Nevertheless, whilst other medical systems may be more in line with local world-views, this does not of itself imply denial of the value of allopathic medicine.

In Rajasthan, the protective measures followed are drawn eclectically from the various traditions. The strict dietary rules followed by pregnant women and new mothers, to prevent humoral imbalances and indigestion, come from the Ayurvedic tradition. Connected to the spiritual world, diverse amulets and threads are tied around the child's waist and neck, whilst 'evil eye' is countered with the black marks put on the face of a newborn child. These black marks are called '*tika*', a term adopted by health authorities to designate 'vaccines' in Hindi, although none of our informants made this connection. Astrological charts can show that the child has certain weak spots, which can be countered through rituals or amulets that strengthen certain stars in their birth horoscopes. Spirits and gods need always to be taken care of through rituals or by amulets or through putting a dagger under the child's pillow, lest their anger or jealousy strike a vulnerable child. To a large extent Muslims and Hindus in the Rajasthan field sites use each other's healers, and certain lines from the Muslim holy book, the Qur'an, can also create a protective space for the Hindu child when needed.

All of the above measures are treated as necessary, although they are of different provenance and socioritual importance. Some of the actions, like binding amulets or performing rituals, must be performed by different kinds of experts. Others practices, like deciding what to eat or placing a dagger under a pillow, are common knowledge shared by mothers, mothers-in-laws, and neighbours, and only on rare occasions are herbal experts or Ayurvedic doctors consulted about them. Against this background, government health workers only interfere in the popular dietary rules where the advice of government doctors creates confusion and fears about doing things wrong. Vaccination, on the other hand, does not interfere with but complements popular practice. Vaccination as a medical technology thus operates in a pluralistic medical system where it is one, but not *the,* form of child protection. Numerous people to whom mothers relate actively influence their decisions or give advice: mothers-in-law, husbands, and educated or uneducated neighbours who relate their different experiences, priests and prophets, local healers, and 'doctors' of varying standards of legality and education. Our discussions with young mothers show that they are confused about whose advice to take and lack the money or freedom to explore alternatives. And, as stated above, their experiences with government health facilities are sometimes negative, either in terms of being treated without dignity, or even maltreated, or in terms of not getting better. Consultation sessions with doctors, as with healers, are open to the general public (who are present), and information about affliction, needs, or treatment is kept to a bare minimum. Allopathic medicine/biomedicine is not seen as challenging or conflicting with established popular knowledge of health and the body. How and when people turn to biomedical practitioners depends on many things, although information couched in biomedical terms is rarely found convincing. In Orissa, even when vaccination is accepted, the programme may subsequently fail because of competing needs or commitments, for example during peak agricultural seasons. Vaccination sometimes results in a child experiencing fever and pain. Anxious mothers then start to doubt, and through chatting and gossiping with concerned neighbours begin to spread their scepticism.

Vaccines are products of biomedical science, but vaccination is also a behaviour prescribed by the state, with which citizens are under pressure to comply. Such pressures are manifested in different forms and strategies in our various study settings. For instance, in the Orissa community the state is projected as a benevolent entity that is concerned about the poverty of tribal people, offering them a range of social welfare and development services. Thus we are told that 'we tribal are poor and have so many diseases, the government is providing vaccines so that we survive and don't die of diseases', 'the Government has made a rule that women should deliver in the hospital for which the Government gives us 1400 rupees'. None of them (including the ASHA) knew that such cash is given as an incentive. They rather configured this cash as alms. (In Rajasthan, rather differently, we found that health workers do see it as an incentive which is sought and appreciated. However, because of high rates of under-the-table payments to delivering doctors and nurses, and the risk of other expenses in case of complications, not everybody was sufficiently motivated.) People in Orissa use the money to pay off debts, to open a bank account, to buy a goat (an important asset in tribal communities) or in connection with naming ceremonies. From our discussions it appeared that nobody related it to post-partum care or assistance for transportation for hospital delivery. The 1400 rupees paid as part of the safe motherhood initiative is widely seen as part of larger poverty alleviation measures, and economic vulnerability and poverty are significant factors in generating demand for vaccination.

Other schemes, like the old-age pension scheme or infrastructure provisions, reinforce the benevolent image of the state. Villagers are aware of such schemes and demand these services from the health workers. While population control remains a major drive in these areas, as is mandatory HIV/AIDS testing, this does not negate the state's benevolent image. Health workers are often able to manipulate, negotiate or compromise. In one case the ASHA manipulated the number of children in the delivery record and got away with it. Similarly, the cash incentives provided by the government are sometimes claimed even when women deliver at home or on the way to the hospital. Such negotiations establish the state as a powerful agent, but not necessarily a strict disciplinarian. Also interestingly, it is men more than women who clearly articulate many of these practices as government interventions. 'Vaccines are given by government and it is their job', 'Government knows the diseases and the block office sends people to administer vaccines', 'Government has made rule that we will get 1400 rupees for hospital delivery as the government knows we *adivasi* (aboriginals) don't have the money to eat food and are poor'. The everyday forms of governance come across as subtle but visible.

In Rajasthan, attempts to be a 'good citizen' are articulated through desires to be 'modern'. 'We vaccinate because we are not backward anymore' asserted one Rajasthani village woman. Those stressing their modernity and status were usually higher caste and class people. This kind of statement plays directly into the segmentation of Rajasthani society, and similar caste and class discourse was used to exclude the disadvantaged from being 'good people'. The same individuals saw lack of education as a prime mark of 'dirty people'. In schools, people are taught to trust the government and its agenda of modernisation. Hence, although many said they did not know what vaccines are or do in the body (either in terms of local ideas of protection or in bioscientific terms), they still were proud to say they vaccinate because they are 'educated' or 'not backward'. For most people in these groups, social pressures make it important to say yes to vaccination in order to be a good, modern, and civilized person. However, workers in the health system also used similar language, labelling specific groups as bad citizens or 'dirty people' (see Nordfeldt and Roalkvam 2010). Muslims or tribal groups were especially likely to be labelled as such. Although health workers might make an exception for specific Muslims or tribals, 'Oh, those are good Gurjars' (Gurjars are a Rajasthani ST), they did so without letting it influence their rhetoric or general view about the group (Nordfeldt and Roalkvam 2010).

We observed a strong connection between people's wish to be modern and their following government health advice, and by the same token a strong idea that those who did not follow the advice were backward. This is not so surprising. For decades the Indian government has been engaged in propagating a message of modernity, linking the image of an ideal citizen to a range of national health, population control, and development programmes. According to Singh and Bharadwaj (2000), the mass media strategies on immunisation crafted by the Indian central government during the 1980s and 1990s represent the biggest ever communication and mobilisation programme it has undertaken. Messages of different types were crafted, all attempting to 'forge alliances' between the government and different levels of the population (Singh and Bharadwaj 2000, p. 668). Some typical messages show how immunisation is made part of a moral discourse of modernity and good citizenship. In addition to question-and-answer type messages for more informed segments of the population, simple immunisation messages could be used to address everyone: slogans like 'Be wise, immunise' or 'Be a friend, help eradicate polio' (Singh and Bharadwaj 2000, p. 669). The first appeals to the good judgement of the progressive and educated, the second to a sense of a national community and common fate. The national immunisation programme booklet called *A Pact of Partnership* underlined the duty of the citizen towards the nation to 'act as responsible partners' in order to 'build a better and healthier future for our country' (cited in Singh and Bharadwaj 2000, p. 671). After 1990, the polio eradication campaign stated that '145 countries have done it, INDIA too can do it. Eradicate polio!' (Singh and Bharadwaj 2000, p. 671).

The Indian campaigns and visual imagery were and are linked to messages of family planning in posters and health promotion campaigns. It is the middle-class, well-educated, one-child or two-children family that is portrayed in the health information messages. Both the project of immunisation and the communication strategies are well intended, but when their products travel between communities, their original meanings become entangled with other, perhaps very different, social experiences. Discourses of good citizenship can easily transmute into blame games. As shown above, higher classes and health personnel blame the most vulnerable and mistreated social groups for the problems facing modernisation and development, thereby hindering positive dialogue and information sharing. In information campaigns, the messages of wisdom, of the nation as community and of progress, revert into the implicit discourse of blame when groups or individuals do not act in accordance with official notions of good citizenship.

In the case of Malawi, the health songs seem to fulfil much the same purpose as the Indian campaign slogans. However, the numerous songs were popular, known nationally, often played on the radio, and supported by widespread social usage (Alfsen 2011). In terms of Ong's notion of 'technologies of subjection', Malawi's songs are a much more successful technology than the Indian campaigns, which played a part in convincing some but succeeded only in alienating others.

In Malawi, as in India (although without the class differences so evident in Rajasthan), pressure put on women is linked to broader health and other development initiatives. Here too, vaccination practices are intimately tied to family planning regimes (introduced in 1994 by the late President Dr Banda). Social pressure to comply with biomedical regimes was applied to mothers falling short of these expectations regarding the 'good mother'. Thus, mothers who fail to comply with vaccination regimens, family planning, or norms of cleanliness might experience various forms of social pressure, including rumours of witchcraft. Pressures are intended to induce compliance with social expectations regarding cleanliness and motherhood, but also agricultural activities. After all, a starving family puts a burden on the whole village. In such a social context vaccination represents a moral choice that extends well beyond the relations between mothers and children (cf. Danielsen 2011).

In the Indian context, despite social pressures from the state and society to enhance compliance, agency is often exercised through individual refusals (although in our research we found no instances of collective resistance). Neither trust nor compliance can be taken for granted, and health workers devise individualised strategies to elicit and sustain trust. The most common way of resisting vaccination was to simply not show up, even after agreeing to come during the mobilisation meetings. In the harvest season non-attendance would be explained by saying 'people are too busy', in the hot season, 'the heat could threaten the child'. Even when accepted, vaccines were not always seen as essential. Fever was, however, the reason most commonly given in both Orissa and Rajasthan for not vaccinating (and sometimes in Malawi too). It could be that caretakers were afraid that the fever that can follow vaccination could harm the child. It could also be because they found the child's crying annoying, or that the fever and the crying would disrupt the mother's household and agricultural work.

In one case in Rajasthan, in a village where compliance with the vaccination programme was the accepted norm, there was outright resistance towards the ASHA and ANM following a breach of trust. The health workers lied to young women and their mothers-in-law about the real nature of what they were doing as they inserted IUDs in the young women. The ASHA in this case was put under pressure by the ANM. After this incident, some mothers or grandmothers would take their infants to a nearby town for injections, and some would skip a month of injections. This power-play led to a noticeable protest against the ANMs and ASHA's abuse of trust and power: evidence that the asymmetrical power relationship can be shifted or restructured.

Social pressures are at times visible while at other times they are subtle and have in effect been normalised. As discussed earlier in this book day-to-day vaccine behaviour to a large extent is routinised and follows more from passive acceptance than from any active demand. Mothers in the tribal villages of Orissa say 'we do it as everybody does it'. A similar notion of acceptance as a norm was found to be widespread in Malawi. However, such acceptance–demand dynamics can be disrupted by extraordinary events and situations: whether the vaccine-related rumours we discussed in previous chapters or in Malawi, where the measles outbreak clearly showed active demand emerging in response to a situation that had suddenly become acute.

As the previous section suggests, neither in Malawi nor in India can we understand vaccination response in terms of clear-cut and mutually exclusive categories of acceptance and resistance. Vaccines are actively sought in some cases in Malawi, as shown by mothers' and caretakers' disappointment when HSAs fail to show up with vaccines at an outreach clinic. Such a positive attitude is also shown by the fact that mothers are less interested to continue attending the outreach clinic after the completion of the vaccine schedule, which ends with measles vaccine when the child is 9 months old. As the case study from the outreach clinic in Thyolo shows, mothers who fail to demonstrate children's vaccination through health passports or cards face ridicule, social sanctions, and challenges in accessing other health services for their children. Because proof of vaccination is important, and sought by the health workers, mothers are willingly compliant. Thus the evidence in all the three contexts shows that demand for vaccination at the community level is a complex phenomenon. Community demand may have a variety of sources. It may represent a normalised acceptance (as everybody does it, so do we). It may be that vaccine acceptance is the compromise required in order to meet more pressing demands: for curative medicines for example, or following from starvation or malnutrition. Acceptance of vaccine may reflect a desire to appear modern or it may be the result of reciprocal social obligations. All these connotations must be situated in the larger context of vaccine delivery. Vaccination is never simply about the practical procurement and 'delivery' of vaccines. The sociocultural and political context plays a crucial role and cannot be seen merely as 'interference' or the cause of failure and misunderstanding. How precisely vaccines are delivered is significant for understanding behaviour: processes of compliance, adherence or reinterpretation. It makes a difference, for example, if they are free or not; provided on a fixed day in the village or not, whether or not through a health passport conceived of as a 'ticket' to accessing other state services, and whether or not vaccination is combined with other services. How vaccination fits with other elements of popular knowledge regarding child protection is also critical. Community demand, and thus vaccine coverage—and most importantly its longer term sustainability—depends on all these factors.

Conclusions

Ethnographic evidence from the three regions studied shows how deeply implicated immunisation practices are in a range of contexts and processes, both political and sociocultural. To understand how and why immunisation coverage can be high or uneven in different contexts it is necessary to understand how governance works: the role of the chief in Malawi, for example, or the ways in which the performance of health workers is monitored and controlled. It is necessary to understand the mode of delivering vaccines as well as the strategies and mechanisms with which health workers handle the competing pressures of meeting targets and eliciting the trust of the community.

In this chapter we hope to have shown how vaccination as a biomedical, but also as a government, intervention is located in a range of health practices (beginning with local child health protective practices) and engagements (with health workers and the services they can offer, the strategies they employ, but also with the state, as 'poor tribal people' or 'good modern citizens'). It is the actual operation of such fragile mechanisms, dependent as they are on the larger economic and political context of a region, that result in consistently high coverage in one place and variations over time in another. In many parts of the world response to vaccination has little to do with epidemiological proofs of the merits of a vaccine or with biomedical explanations of immunity. Rather, it is embedded in a host of other larger economic, political, and social factors, the structure of local society, and the ways in which a host of actors (health workers of various kinds, local chiefs in Malawi, other healers, members of the family and neighbourhood, and so on) interact with each other. It is the interplay of such actors, contexts, and processes that helps us understand why there could be high and sustained immunisation coverage rate in Malawi while, despite widespread acceptance of immunisation in a tribal community in Orissa, the number of *fully* immunised children could be much lower. Even when vaccines are accepted or sought, a programme may appear to be failing.

Chapter 7

Have means become ends? Getting children's health back in focus

Stuart Blume, Sidsel Roalkvam, and Desmond McNeill

Introduction

Modern vaccines are among the most powerful tools available to public health. They have saved millions of lives, protected millions more against the ravages of crippling and debilitating disease, and have the capacity to save many millions more. But like all complex and sophisticated tools, they can be used for different purposes, in different ways, and with various consequences. This seems strange. Surely, vaccines can and should be used for one sole purpose: to protect children against the risks to their health of vaccine-preventable diseases? A brief reflection on the history of vaccination shows that this is far too simple. When polio eradication was proposed as a global objective, in the late 1980s, it was vigorously debated. No one doubted the power of the polio vaccine to protect children. But experts differed in how they thought it should best be used. There have been some who have regarded vaccination programmes as a means of strengthening primary health care, whilst others have seen them as likely to divert attention and resources from needed improvements in health services. At issue in such debates is not the immunological properties of a vaccine, but the way in which it should best be used. Taking the healthcare needs of children, and especially those whose health is most at risk, as the key objective, how should vaccines best be deployed? Neither public health officials nor front-line health workers have the time or the inclination to pose such a question. They try to do their best with the tools they have, given the pressures and the constraints under which they have to work.

In a recent contribution to the debate on the future of the British National Health Service, historian of science and medicine John Pickstone pointed to an intriguing contradiction (Pickstone 2011). Britain has long been committed to grounding decisions regarding the introduction of new procedures or treatments on a strong evidential base. Also, new forms of consultation, of involving patients in evaluating the benefits of new treatments, have been pioneered in Britain. In other words, when a new drug is made available in the health service, there should be reasonable confidence in its safety, (cost) effectiveness, and acceptability to patients. How different, argues Pickstone, when it comes to the overall functioning and organisation of the health services within which these treatments are provided. Decisions about the health service as a whole, how it should be (re)organised and funded, have been based wholly on ideological predispositions, without recourse to empirical evidence. This provocative argument implies a distinction between a realm of technical, evidence-based decision-making, and one governed by ideological commitments to, for example, market forces, privatisation, and the decentralisation of health service governance. Although this book is concerned mainly with countries in the south, Pickstone's argument is relevant, raising as it does such central issues as the role of evidence in decision-making, the involvement of patients and, more generally, the power of ideology.

This book has focused on a particular set of technologies—vaccines—and on the rules, institutions, and practices through which they are put to use. On the one hand new vaccines are subjected to long, expensive, multisited trials designed to establish their safety, efficacy, duration of protection, and so on. On the other hand, strategic decisions, which have shaped the overall immunisation system, have not been based on such rigorous testing and debate. Following William Muraskin, it was argued in Chapter 1, for example, that the beginnings of the polio eradication campaign derived from the unshakeable commitment of a small group of experts to the notion of eradication. This is not to say that evidence played no part. But evidence, like experience, can be interpreted in different ways. The success of the global smallpox eradication campaign was used to justify a follow-up campaign targeting another disease (in the event, polio). Some, including the Director General of WHO, felt that this was not the correct conclusion to be drawn from the smallpox campaign.

This example is less unusual than it seems. Values, interests, and prior experience shape the ways in which evidence is interpreted (or 'framed') and the actions based on those interpretations. In the early 1960s it first became clear that the oral polio vaccine (OPV), which had been almost universally preferred to Salk's inactivated vaccine (IPV), occasionally became virulent. A number of cases of vaccine-induced poliomyelitis were identified. There was then epidemiological evidence for a very small, but real, risk associated with the vaccine, which was not the case with IPV. Weighing the relative merits of the two vaccines necessarily involved political judgments in which questions such as public confidence in the vaccine, cost, and vaccine availability all played their part. In the event the USA, and most other countries, continued using OPV exclusively until the 1990s (Blume 2005). Contrast this with the events surrounding the rotavirus vaccine RotaShield. A year after the vaccine had been licensed in the USA (1998), by which time it was already in widespread use, a small number of cases of intussusception were discovered and attributed to the vaccine. Its manufacturer immediately withdrew it from the market even though at that time no alternative vaccine was available. Of course there were great differences in popular anxieties regarding the two diseases in the USA. Unlike polio in the 1960s, rotavirus infection in the USA is rarely fatal and was scarcely a 'dread disease'. In developing countries, where rotavirus infection often is fatal, the small risk of intussusception might have weighed less heavily with decision-makers. But withdrawal of the vaccine pre-empted any such assessment. The contrasting responses in the USA show the influence of changing social values, and of changes in the acceptability of risk over this 30-year period.

In trying to address the question 'How can vaccines best be used in the interests of children's health?' this book has attempted to subject to critical scrutiny the values, the assumptions, and the reasoning underlying the functioning of vaccination programmes. This is the kind of thing that social scientists regularly do, and we have made use largely of concepts, perspectives, and modes of investigation drawn from the social sciences. The result is an analysis somewhat different from what is usual in public health. We have not looked at immunisation practices from the point of view of the physician or the epidemiologist, and have avoided assuming that there is one 'right' way of doing things. There is no privileged position from which one can understand all the values, beliefs, pressures, and trade-offs that shape decisions, whether those of a mother or those of a Minister of Health. We have attempted to analyse both 'positive' decisions (vaccine adoption or acceptance) and 'negative' decisions (non-adoption or vaccine rejection), and the processes and logics underlying those decisions. What are the assumptions, and particularly the implicit taken-for-granted assumptions, on which the system seems in practice to rest? How far, and in what ways, are these assumptions problematic? Two things will become apparent in this final chapter. One is that there is nothing fixed or inevitable about these assumptions. As suggested in Chapter 1, they evolve over time, in response to changes in the relative influence and authority of the various stakeholders involved in formulating them. For example, encouraging the introduction of new vaccines into national immunisation schedules became a global objective in the late 1980s. Assumptions and objectives evolve in response to the opportunities that new technology brings with it, but also in response to changes in the interests and the ideology that dominate political processes. Objectives or assumptions that were once questionable, and were questioned, may gradually come to seem self-evident. Investments—of money, but also of reputation—grow to such an extent that 'there's no turning back now', and debate dies down. But the fact remains that the objectives and assumption on which global public health today rests, whether debated or not, are the product of specific configurations of interests and ideologies. This is not to say that policies do not need to be justified and actors called to account.

A second focus of this chapter will be on how and to whom decisions are justified. With what kind of argument, with appeals to what kind of evidence, are actions justified? And to whom are those taking the decisions accountable? This may sound like a question more suited to a book on political theory than one on public health, but it is in fact central to understanding what goes on at the various interfaces discussed in the book. With what arguments does an MoH justify its decision to introduce, or not to introduce, a new vaccine? It is not too difficult to think of some of the arguments to which an MoH could appeal: cost, epidemiological data (or their lack), the advice of WHO experts, long-term sustainability or the experience of a neighbouring country. But a more challenging question follows. To whom, when, and where is an MoH *obliged* to justify its actions? This is another way of asking: to whom or what are governments accountable? The kind of arguments that will provide an acceptable justification depend on whom, or what organisation, has to be satisfied. This is just as true of a mother who has decided to have her child vaccinated, or not to have her child vaccinated. How does she explain her decision? By referring to the costs or difficulties in getting the vaccination done? By appealing to her trust in the doctor or nurse or health worker, or her lack of trust? Or that the child already had a vaccination and surely that's enough, or perhaps that this is a disease better prevented in other, traditional, ways. Here too the important question follows. Where and to whom is that mother obliged to justify her decision? A decision not to vaccinate may have to be justified to an angry health worker, whether in a village in Malawi or a children's health centre in the Netherlands. In the USA, where vaccination is commonly required for admission to a public school, it may have to be justified in a court of law. Questions relating to the kind of evidence and the kinds of arguments that are used to justify courses of action, and to whom (accountability), are crucial to understanding the functioning of the immunisation system as analysed in this book.

Goals and targets

One of the trends identified in Chapter 1 was that global goals and targets have been key to the evolution of programmes from the beginnings of EPI onwards. Why do global goals and targets figure so prominently? And where are their effects felt? Only at the level of the state, or do they filter down to that of the community-based health worker?

The prominence of global goals and targets in discussing the effectiveness of immunisation programmes is the result of two related but analytically distinguishable developments.

For many years health-related work in developing countries was referred to as international health. 'International health' referred to an international field of engaged nation states, and development and health institutions. During the last decade we have seen a gradual replacing of the term 'international health' with 'global health'. Various scholars have commented on this transition: on how it came about, what it signifies, and what its consequences might be. All agree that more than mere semantics is involved (e.g. Fidler 2004; Brown et al. 2006; Koplan et al. 2009; Brada 2011). For some, a world of vastly enhanced mobility, the increasingly permeable nature of national boundaries, and the ease and the speed with which epidemics spread mean that national responses can no longer be adequate, so that control of infectious disease is only possible in the context of globally coordinated action. Other writers look more critically at what is done, and what is not done, where and to whom, in the name of global health. For some critics, 'global health' stands for the ways in which the north engages with the health problems of communities in the global south that lack the expertise and the resources to deal with them (Brada 2011). Only in this way, by putting the sophisticated tools of western technology in place, can northern countries protect themselves against the dangers arising in these distant breeding grounds of disease.

Whichever terminology, and hence perspective, one prefers, the concept of 'global health' has become self-evident. Few, today, find anything strange in the notion of a 'global immunisation strategy', or the 'Global Vaccines Action Plan' that followed Bill Gates' proposal at the 2010 World Economic Forum. Initiatives like these seem justifiable, at the very least, because the notion of public health as a necessarily global concern is, broadly speaking, taken for granted.

Within the new sphere of 'global public health' that has come into being over the past two or three decades, a variety of institutions jockey for position; sometimes collaborating, sometimes competing for influence and resources. Chapter 3 argued that the activities of these various institutions can (and do) draw on various sources of authority: WHO's mandate, and its accountability to the WHA, give it formal legal authority. The World Bank, by contrast, derives its influence mainly from the financial resources it controls. To these were added moral authority and expertise, both of which are relevant to UNICEF. Especially important, however, is what was termed 'performance legitimacy', typically attributed to the business sector. Among these various forms of authority today one, money, has become more powerful than the rest. And among the variety of global institutions concerned with immunisation the GAVI Alliance has become the most significant, not only because of the coherence and coordination it was able to bring to the field, but also because of the funds it has at its disposal. Today, a large share of the resources that WHO can devote to immunisation come from GAVI, whilst many donor countries have chosen to channel their immunisation-related aid through GAVI. The Alliance defines itself principally by reference to its commitment to the introduction of new vaccines. At the time of writing, GAVI's home page proudly announces that Zimbabwe has introduced pneumococcal vaccine, Yemen the rotavirus vaccine, North Korea the pentavalent vaccine, and Ghana 'two new vaccines at once'.

The other fundamental change that underpins today's emphasis on goals and targets results from an increasing pressure from donor countries for aid, in all sectors, to be results-based, in the name of 'development effectiveness'. Today, despite continuing or even increased talk of 'country ownership', there are growing demands for performance accountability, reflected in demands for measurement of performance—not just outputs, but also outcomes and impacts—based on objective quantitative indicators. The MDGs have contributed to the process. One of the attractions of vaccines is precisely their measurability: as regards both specifying targets and measuring achievement. Dividing the number of vaccines distributed by the number of children of the appropriate age in the target population is made to yield two simple but powerful numbers: percentage coverage and number of lives saved. Formulating simple and realisable objectives in terms of quantifiable targets that would appeal to donors, and hence facilitating the mobilisation of resources, has been central to the global programmes discussed in this book. The appeal of the MDGs, and their success in mobilising political and financial support, is partly due to a successful reframing of poverty—and of ill health as one manifestation of it—within a new landscape of risks, responsibilities, and opportunities. Infectious disease is seen as a threat not only to an individual person, but to the economy, to development, and to stability. The MDGs were expressed in a language that presented poverty and ill health as challenges that could be alleviated by a combination of money and technology, and a commitment on the part of western countries to supplying them. The global community was willing to support these goals largely because they were convinced by the rationale of evidence-based and cost-effective measures justified by an explicit economic rationale. The MDGs were very successful in mobilising resources from donors, but they have also defined an incentive structure—based on results-based management—holding governments and donors to account on delivery against the MDG benchmarks (Sumner and Lawo 2010). The focus tends to be on the 'we' who are to save 'them' (the poor). This distracts attention from what is actually going on in one country or another. The sites of intervention provide the décor against which the moral drama can be played out.

The logic underlying the succession of global immunisation goals and programmes that followed on from smallpox eradication is essentially that of international politics. Each programme was crafted in the light of the balance of political interests of its time, inflected with the dominant ideology of its time, and with the need to mobilise resources and sustain donor commitments always central. The growing concern with mobilising resources (as development assistance attracts increasing criticism in many traditional donor countries) and gaining the attention of world political leaders has led to a focus on a few simple attainable goals. The pressure to achieve these goals does not stop at the level of national government. It is transmitted through and down the chain. In Chapter 6 it was argued that the data on immunisation coverage, generated at the village level, 'are not only used as a proxy for health system performance' but 'also used as performance indicators for the village-level health workers'. Just as governments are criticised or rewarded for their performance, so too village-level health workers are evaluated on the basis of numbers: children vaccinated or women registered for antenatal care. The information from Malawi presented in Chapter 6 showed that health workers are not only under pressure to meet targets but also to record data for and report to a range of different health programmes. As a result, according to several informants, health workers felt under pressure to report the numbers that were expected. The risk, otherwise, was that they could lose their jobs. Pressures transmitted through the system, in other words, make the data unreliable.

Incentives and pressures

In the immunisation field there is an expectation that each set of actors along the vaccine chain, from national governments to health workers in the community, will work in accordance with global targets and objectives. What induces them to do so? William Muraskin has pointed out that this does not happen of its own accord. In his words: 'countries as a group have had to be wooed, "educated," and financially enticed to accept the GAVI's goals as their own' (Muraskin 2004, p. 1923). As the quotation implies, this is done through a mixture of financial incentives and more subtle processes of influence.

The more dependent a country is on external funding for maintenance of its health system, the more vital it becomes to keep donors happy, and according to WHO estimates 23 countries have over 30% of their health budgets financed by donors. Malawi is seen by donors as a 'model country' in part because of its high vaccine coverage. This is a source of national pride, but it is an achievement that is heavily dependent on external funds. The costs of failing to conform with global priorities, in other words, are potentially very high indeed. Like goals and targets, financial incentives also work right down through the system. Chapter 6 showed village-level health workers in India being offered rewards for good performance. For mothers too there may be cash incentives. However, financial incentives are not the only instruments with which conformity is produced. Incentives of quite other kinds also permeate the system.

A lack of expertise as well as financial resources makes the governments of poor countries dependent on donors, and incentives may take the form of free advice (where a donor feels that the country concerned lacks the necessary expertise or simply the requisite human resources). Thus a consultant might be paid by GAVI to prepare a request to GAVI on behalf of some country. The latter might indeed be keen to have GAVI support, and simply lack the knowledge or resources needed in order to prepare a satisfactory proposal. But it is also possible that such assistance distorts priorities—since there may be no similar support available to the country wishing to prepare other requests. However, it is not only poor donor-dependent countries, or those lacking technically skilled personnel, that face pressures to conform. It is worth reflecting on the history of vaccine policy in the Netherlands, a small, rich country with an extremely effective national immunisation programme and (until very recently) able to develop and produce vaccines in the public sector. Even here, from the 1980s onwards, developing an immunisation programme on the basis of specifically national assessments of need became increasingly difficult, as pointed out in Chapter 4.

So what are the subtle pressures that ensure that even countries with the financial resources and the expertise to develop and implement their own policies in fact conform to global guidelines and priorities? Part of the answer can be found in political economy and the working of the vaccine industry. From the 1980s until quite recently the industry was marked by growing concentration: a smaller and smaller number of multinational corporations competing in increasingly global markets. Given the huge costs of developing new vaccines, these corporations had (and have) a clear interest in standardisation. Offering the same combination of antigens, to be used according to a common schedule, in all regions and countries makes obvious economic sense. But this is not the only reason why countries conform. Another is conceptual: the concepts with which policy-makers (and the experts who advise them) think about public health, and about how responsibilities are (to be) shared and distributed. We are brought back to the notion of global health. The discursive shift from 'international health' to 'global health' carries with it the idea that public health problems can only be solved at the global level, and that national perspectives have to be subordinated to global consensus. In so doing, in effect, this undermines the rationality, and the legitimacy, of national policy.

Today, more than ever, GAVI (and donors in general) require 'evidence' in quantitative form in order to justify their expenditure. So what are the numbers that count in establishing not only progress but, just as importantly, need? The question of 'what numbers count' is closely connected to another: to whom or what are governments accountable?

Evidence

All policy these days is supposed to be 'evidence-based'. Before a new vaccine is licensed in the USA or Europe comprehensive evidence for its safety and efficacy has to be provided to the regulatory agency. The fragments of vaccine history presented in this book show that where an effective system for reporting adverse events exists, it can generate new evidence leading to reassessment of safety or the duration of protection. This is what happened with RotaShield, which its manufacturer subsequently withdrew from the market. In much of the world, however, adverse event reporting systems do not exist. The question then is, what evidence is collected and what evidence counts? What kinds of data are accepted as providing sufficient proof of safety, or efficacy, or of disease burden? This begs the crucial question of 'Accepted by whom?' There are now various studies, for example of drug regulation, showing that evidence of safety or efficacy found convincing in one forum may be deemed insufficient or unconvincing in another (e.g. Abrahams 2002). So who has to be convinced, and what evidence will they accept? More specifically, since put like that the question is too large to be dealt with fully here, where should that evidence have come from? Does the data have to be national, or will data from somewhere else—anywhere else—on the globe suffice?

There could be biomedical reasons for questioning the applicability of data obtained in a very different environment. The epidemiology of a disease could be quite different, whether as a result of environmental conditions, or the nutritional status of children, or because the pathogen strains circulating differ from those contained in a vaccine. For these reasons, when WHO recommended use of the new rotavirus vaccines in the Americas and in Europe, in 2007, it withheld any recommendation for African and Asian countries until trials there had been completed. Or consider the example of immunisation against measles, as discussed in Chapter 5. It is known that the measles vaccine is safe and effective, but only 80% protective after a single dose. The vaccine should be given when maternal antibodies circulating in infants are too low to offer protection yet not high enough to interfere with the effect of the vaccine. In low-income tropical countries, the intensity of exposure to measles virus is higher and maternal antibodies decline more rapidly than in temperate countries, so that infants are at risk of acquiring measles at a younger age. There are thus good epidemiological reasons for following a measles vaccination schedule different from that employed in northern countries. But since the studies needed in order to establish the optimum schedule are demanding and costly, low-income countries like Malawi are obliged to make use of evidence from other countries (in fact measles vaccination is performed at 9 months of age in many tropical countries).

On behalf of the CVI, Judith Justice found in 1999 that local evidence and the fit with national needs and priorities (including competing priorities within the health sector) played an important role for countries when considering adopting new vaccines (Justice 2000). Neither WHO nor UNICEF was actively promoting new vaccines at that time. It was recognised that new vaccine introduction could threaten weak health systems. Today national data seem to be of declining significance. Policy-makers in a number of countries appear to agree that policy options based on national research are no match for policies based on international research and promoted internationally. This can have unforeseen consequences. One study concluded that 'importing evidence based policies derived in settings outside their own country undermines national experts' experiential knowledge and the credibility of locally-generated solutions' (Behague et al. 2009, p. 1543). The policy-makers in this study came from five countries in which the implementation of new programmes depended on financial support from international donors. In the case of vaccine introduction, at least, something similar seems to be true for richer countries too: the scope for developing nationally specific policies based on local assessments of need is being eroded.

The Indian public health activists discussed in Chapter 4 argued that the government and public sector should establish a strong justification for immunisation through an evidence-based vaccine policy, making their decisions independent of global pressures and commercial interests. The concern was about what is best for the population, from both medical and social perspectives (Madhavi et al. 2010). The public health activists argued that when introduction of pentavalent vaccine was being considered the government advisory body (NTAGI) overlooked evidence for the low incidence of Hib-invasive disease in the Indian population. Criticism here parallels and builds on an earlier critique of the introduction of hepatitis B vaccine starting in 2002 (Madhavi 2003). Here too, according to activist critics, the decision to introduce the vaccine had been based on external pressure, and the interests of the country's biotech industry, rather than on epidemiological evidence from India itself, which did not exist at the time. The Indian public health activists emphasise that they are not 'antivaccine'. They endorse vaccines as a preventive medical tool. Their arguments are that policy must be based on epidemiological data collected in India, and that vaccination must not be a substitute for other basic health measures such as safe drinking water and nutrition (Madhavi et al. 2010).

India has a proud tradition of democratic politics, an active civil society, and substantial and widespread expertise in all the public health-related disciplines. It also has one of the world's most rapidly growing economies, and a strong and growing domestic vaccine industry. The actions of the Indian public health activists have to be seen in the light of the country's traditions, resources, and international standing. The arguments are not only about which numbers are most relevant for vaccine policy. More fundamentally they are about politics and accountability: an insistence that in its public health policy the government should be accountable to the people, and not just to global institutions.

A study of health policy-making in Uganda (discussed in Chapter 2) found that the MoH in that country had become tightly connected to the global public health community, but disconnected from its own local communities. Highly technocratic approaches run deepest in aid-dependent countries. As previous chapters have shown, countries highly dependent on multilateral donors in financing health show a high level of policy capture by global institutions, distorting structures of accountability. Governments become more answerable to donors and multilateral agencies than to the country's representative institutions and the public at large. The local people, in resource-poor settings, are not only sidelined in decisions that affect their lives, the knowledge that they have about life well-lived under difficult circumstances remains a resource not utilised. The same, of course, can be said of the health workers, who form a bridge between the state and the local community.

Health workers are under pressure to report good performance to show that targets are being met. The problems they face, how they balance multiple responsibilities, how they mobilise communities that may be mistrustful or hold very different views regarding health and illness: this kind of knowledge does not travel back up the chain.

Critique is not new

Disputes regarding immunisation policies and practices have always rested on divergent political values. Nineteenth century western European opposition to smallpox vaccination was often rooted in political cleavages in society, in a sense that 'they' were doing things to 'us' largely for 'their' own benefit.

The debates about alternative public health strategies and about disease eradication that took place in Geneva in the 1950s, 1960s and 1970s were suffused with the Cold War politics of the time. The resistance to polio vaccination that emerged in northern Nigeria in 2003 reflected longstanding political tensions between the ethnic groups living in the north and the south of the country. The reason why political discontents are projected onto vaccines and immunisation programmes, as we have pointed out a number of times, is that for many people immunisation symbolises the intrusion of the state, and of supranational institutions, into the most personal of spheres. As Chapter 6 demonstrated, responses of different communities to immunisation reflect the different notions of modernity and of citizenship to be found there, different patterns of social stratification, and different memories of how they had been treated in the past by prevailing powers.

As others (e.g. Leach and Fairhead 2005) have pointed out, public health commentators who attribute parental doubts to ignorance and misinformation are missing the point. Vaccine doubts and anxieties are more importantly about individual autonomy, responsibilities, citizenship, the legitimacy of state action, the influence of multinational corporations, and the market: in short, the things that vaccines and immunisation programmes are seen as signifying. The criticism that the initiatives discussed in this book have attracted has not been about the immunological properties of vaccines; it has been about the ways in which they are deployed, and the grounds on which decisions to use them in one way or another are taken, the factors taken into account or left out of consideration.

Three sets of arguments have surfaced repeatedly in one form or another over the past 30 years.

The numbers are wrong

A decade ago Das et al. (2000) questioned the picture given by standard immunisation-related indicators. The picture was inadequate and misleading, in part because of the pressures on local health workers, the primary source of data. Community-level health workers were inadequately trained to identify vaccine-preventable diseases and failed to record them. Nor were they encouraged to record or report adverse reactions to vaccines. But the inadequacies of the numbers were not due only to failures at the local level. Part of the problem was the way in which international politics led to certain kinds of numbers being emphasised. The conventional practice in reporting coverage, based on the number of doses of various antigens health workers report having distributed and the estimated number of children in the population, is simply inadequate and misleading. Reports of success—such as '80% of the world's children have been immunised and our task is now to reach the remaining 20%'—are based on such misinformation. In their studies of Indian communities they found large numbers of only partially immunised children, even in areas reporting high coverage.

The numbers circulating, quoted in policy documents and debates, are imbued with politics. They reflect prevailing priorities and dominant patterns of accountability. Small wonder that the meaningfulness of the numbers has been the subject of sustained critique. For those committed to primary health care, a high level of immunisation coverage was never going to be an appropriate measure of progress. The criteria against which progress had to be judged were the overall adequacy of the healthcare system, popular satisfaction with that system, and community influence over it (e.g. Newell 1988). Whether one regards as more important the fact of progress towards the MDGs or the fact that such progress could be concealing growing health inequalities (Moser et al. 2005) is unavoidably a matter of political judgement.

'Vertical' programmes such as immunisation undermine health systems

The early years of EPI were marked by ideological conflict over 'vertical' and 'horizontal' approaches to health care. Were development and expansion of the immunisation programme compatible with (or even a means of) strengthening primary health care or an alternative, a betrayal of Alma-Ata ideals, as critics claimed? Despite the heat of those early exchanges, immunisation programmes were not fundamentally either 'vertical' or 'horizontal' (Mills 1983). The rhetoric with which they were explained and justified, and with which resources were mobilised, presented them as one or the other, depending on circumstances. For some, on some occasions, they were to be an essential element in the strengthening of basic healthcare provision, whilst for others, or on other occasions, they would only divert attention from the structural causes of ill health and health inequality. More importantly, there is good reason for believing that the impact of immunisation programmes varies from one place to another. For example, as Taylor et al. discovered, there were significant differences in the effects of the polio eradication campaign, and EPI, on middle-income Latin American countries with well-organised health systems on the one hand, and poor countries with weakly organised health systems on the other (Taylor et al. 1997). The effects were positive in middle-income countries with well-functioning health systems, but in poor countries there was a risk that targeted, vertical immunisation programmes would drain resources from other, routine, health services. So the question is not whether immunisation programmes strengthen or weaken basic health services, but the conditions under which they have one effect or the other. And following on from this, how these effects come about.

In particular, we have to consider how vaccines reach communities: the reliability of their arrival, their 'packaging' with other (perhaps more actively desired) services, the involvement of health workers delivering vaccinations in the local communities they serve. Immunisation programmes can enhance both demand for health services and their accessibility. Or they can have the opposite effect. The right kind of 'packaging' makes it easier for health workers to motivate the community. The material benefits attaching to some services (for example the cash payments Indian families receive for institutional delivery) are used by health workers in the Indian context to generate not only compliance with vaccination but overall trust in their services.

There is no (single) answer to the question of whether immunisation programmes strengthen health services or undermine them. It depends on budgetary processes in MoHs, on the robustness of health services, and also on the way in which immunisation is combined with other services and the way health workers at the front line manage their multiple responsibilities.

Programmes are not sustainable

Even if immunisation programmes don't by definition undermine basic health care, the programmes as they are now run are not sustainable. Governments of poor countries will be neither willing nor able to pay for them once donor support ends. There is some evidence for this. Chapter 1 quoted from a study of the impact of a vertical immunisation programme established in Ecuador in the 1980s with support from USAID (Gloyd et al. 2003). The researchers found that the vast investment in NIDs had had a significant short-term, but little long-term, effect. When support from USAID ended, both administrative organisation and routine programmes had difficulty in filling the gap created. Immediately after the intensive immunisation programmes ended numbers of measles cases rose to higher levels than they had been before the programmes started.

The answer, according to researchers who have worked in local communities, is to design programmes corresponding to what people actually want. The anthropologist Mark Nichter thus distinguished between 'active demand' for a vaccine and its 'passive acceptance' (Nichter 1995). By the former he meant 'adherence to vaccination programs by an informed public which perceives the benefits of and need for specific vaccinations'. If vaccination programmes are to be sustainable, Nichter argued, the focus has to be on enhancement of 'community demand', not increased coverage rate. The tendency to assume that once high coverage had been achieved people would see the benefits was not supported by community-level studies.

Critiques of numbers, verticality, and sustainability are far from new, but they seem to have had rather little impact on global health policy. The main reason, we suggest, is that which we identified earlier, when referring to what Pickstone wrote about the British NHS: it is a matter of ideology. What is at stake in this case is not so much belief in neo-liberalism and the market, as a more benign yet no less powerful belief—in a top-down, target-and-performance-based approach. Global support for immunisation, massive when measured in money terms, focuses mainly on the supply side. To be sure, this powerful ideology is combined with moral commitment to saving children's lives. In such circumstances those who ask critical questions are not easily heard. There is no doubt that global immunisation programmes have great achievements to their credit, but it seems that mobilising resources and 'keeping health on the agenda' have become ends in themselves. Strategic considerations, supported by ideological convictions and bolstered by good moral arguments, are now leading to a growing convergence of health and foreign policy. Dealing with the developing world's diseases has become a key feature of many nations' foreign policies. There seem good reasons for believing that this not only creates growing mistrust between nations (Rushton 2011), but takes 'health' further and further from people. Health can be understood as the strength to be human: to make use of one's physical and mental capacities, to practice freedoms. As the anthropologist Veena Das put it some years ago: 'we have to see how we may define health so that instead of becoming a . . . means by which power may be exercised upon the one who declares that he is in pain, it becomes a means for the practices of freedom' (Das 1989, p. 43). If the focus of 'global health' is to be 'health', rather than minimising threat or deploying technology, then attention surely has to be redirected towards those who seek health for themselves and their children, and to the relations and structures that support or inhibit them in their search. To say this is not to deny the crucial role that vaccines, both old and new, have to play. It is, however, to question the programmes, structures, and (ultimately) ideologies that now shape their use.

What is to be done?

For immunisation systems to function, trust is crucial: trust in vaccines, trust in the professionals who administer them, trust in the government and the health system under which those professionals work. But it cannot be taken for granted. Trust can suddenly be broken by the outbreak of an epidemic or by the emergence (or resurgence) of political tensions, but it can only be built up slowly, and for the most part it is the health workers in the community who build and sustain trust: the ASHAs and ANMs in India, the HSAs in Malawi, and their equivalents elsewhere. The pressures under which health workers in poor countries have to work, and the incentive structure to which they must respond, do not encourage the creation of trust. Nor do they encourage the creation of active community demand for vaccines. Building trust appears rather to be a matter for personal initiative. Many health workers are successful in this, but it is not supported by the system many of them work in. Required to report almost exclusively on short-term coverage targets, health workers have an incentive to exaggerate performance and are unwilling to report fundamental health problems (such as malnutrition or low birth weights) because their superiors will interpret such reports as a sign of their having failed.

The same is true of vaccine-related adverse events: an important indicator of vaccine safety, cold chain weakness or some other failure. Parents in the industrialised world often have access to compensation schemes in the event of vaccine failure, which offers reassurance and helps breed trust. In much of the world there is no system for identifying such events, and health workers face disincentives to reporting on them. Here too any such report will be interpreted in terms of their personal failure. The lack of a system for reporting what, to a community, appears as a clear instance of vaccine failure has implications which seem not to be appreciated. The emergence of rumour and of collective resistance, for example as occurred with the pilot HPV vaccine project in India, surely feed on the absence of institutionalised mechanisms for investigating and reporting suspicions arising in the community.

Reporting systems, surveillance systems, incentive structures driving the collection of local data: all are designed principally to reassure donors and global institutions that their plans are being implemented and targets are being achieved, but such systems and structures suppress knowledge of the local realities under which health workers work and communities live.

Philippe Calain has argued that the most important function of surveillance systems should be empowerment of front-line healthcare providers (Calain 2006a). But if surveillance data are to be meaningful and reliable, an incentive structure that encourages accurate reporting has to be crafted. This applies not only to health workers, but to communities too: 'communities can only be motivated to report on unusual events by the reward of free, accessible health care . . . initiatives to fund surveillance programmes cannot work in abstraction from overall deficiencies of health systems' (Calain 2006a).

What is to be done? The answer, we suggest, is to take the notion of 'evidence-based policy' seriously; to interpret evidence more widely than mere numbers, to include knowledge of, and about, the local community. The proper scope of such data will not necessarily be limited to what has been usual in epidemiology. For example, Das et al. argued that policy should be informed by studies focusing on the characteristics of communities, not households, or individuals (Das et al. 2000). No less important, it is with such data that governments can best explain and justify their priorities and choices to their citizens. Strengthening the data collection, research, and analytic capacities of public health authorities in this direction will facilitate renewal of the accountability of governments to their citizens: an accountability that is in danger of being severely compromised.

In the new field of public health ethics a good deal of attention is devoted to constraints on individual behaviour that are justified by appeals to the common good. In recent years, fears of a major threat to the health (and hence the security) of the nation have been used to justify coercions and restrictions of many kinds. And whilst fear of bioterrorism is an extreme instance, it seems that 'global public health' in general—and immunisation as one of its most effective tools—is slowly moving in the direction of securitisation. Unlike 'populations'—the numbers on the basis of which coverage can be calculated—citizens have rights. One of those rights, in democratic societies, is to hold government accountable for its actions. If this is to be as true for public health as it for educational policy, or fiscal or industrial policy, then the implications need to be spelled out clearly. We would like to see immunisation programmes rescued from the strategic interests that have come to define global health. We would like to see them not just 'evidence-based', but 'knowledge-based', where 'knowledge' includes acknowledgement of the relevance of wisdom born of living in a particular community, culture or environment. We would like to see immunisation programmes in poor countries (re)integrated into processes of community development. We would like to see the health and well-being of children, rather than the optimum deployment of health technology, as the ultimate measure of progress.

References

Aaby, P. and C.J. Clements (1989). Measles immunization research: a review. *Bulletin of the World Health Organization* 67(4), 443–448.

Abrahams, J. (2002). The pharmaceutical industry as a political player. *The Lancet* 360, 1498–1502.

Adamson, P. (2001). 'The mad American', in R. Jolly (ed.), *Jim Grant. UNICEF visionary*. Florence: Innocenti Research Centre. Available at http://www.unicef irc.org/publications/pdf/jim_grant_book.pdf (accessed 30 October 2012).

Addlakha, R. (2001). State legitimacy and social suffering in a modern epidemic: A case study of dengue haemorrhagic fever in Delhi. *Contributions to Indian Sociology* 35(2), 151–179.

Alfsen, K. (2011). *HSAs and the Wisdom to Handle Knowledge: A Study of Health Surveillance Assistants' work in Rural Malawi*. Master's thesis, Department of Social Anthropology. Oslo: University of Oslo.

Amrith, S.S. (2006). *Decolonizing International Health: India and Southeast Asia, 1930–1965*. London: Palgrave Macmillan.

Amsden, A.H. (2007). *Escape from Empire*. Cambridge, MA: MIT Press.

Arora, N. (2012). *Opportunities for vaccine introduction and identifying knowledge gaps*. Presentation to the meeting of the SAGE 11 April. Session: Impact of introduction of new vaccines on the strengthening of immunization and health systems. Available at http://www.who.int/immunization/sage/meetings/2012/april/3_N.Arora_FinalSAGESession5NUVI_Impact.pdf.

Aylward, R.B. and J. Linkins (2005). Polio eradication: mobilizing and managing the human resources. *Bulletin of the World Health Organization* 83(4), 268–273.

Aylward, R.B, H.F. Hull, S.L. Coch, R.W. Sutter, J.M. Olive, and B. Melgaard (2000). Disease eradication as a public health strategy: a case study of poliomyelitis eradication. *Bulletin of the World Health Organization* 78(3), 285–297.

Babalola, S. and U. Lawan (2009). Factors predicting BCG immunization status in Northern Nigeria: A behavioural and ecological perspective. *Journal of Child Health Care* 14(1), 46–62.

Balarajan, Y., S. Selvarai, and S.V. Subramanian (2011). Health care and equity in India. *The Lancet* 377(9764), 505–515.

Banerjee, A. and E. Duflo (2011). *Poor Economics. A Radical Rethinking of the Way to Fight Global Poverty*. New York: Public Affairs Press.

Banerji, D. (1984) Primary health care: selective or comprehensive? *World Health Forum* 5, 312–315.

Barnett, M. and M. Finnemore (2004). *Rules for the World: International Organizations In Global Politics*. Ithaca: Cornell University Press.

Barrett, S. (2007). *Why Cooperate: The Incentive to Supply Global Public Goods*. New York: Oxford University Press.

Basch, P.F. (1994). *Vaccines and World Health. Science, Policy, and Practice*. New York and Oxford: Oxford University Press.

Batniji, R. and E. Bendavid (2012). Does development assistance for health really displace government health spending? Reassessing the evidence. *PloS Medicine* 9(5), e1001214. doi:10.1371/journal.pmed.1001214. Available at http://www.plosmedicine.org/article/info%3Adoi%2F10.1371%2Fjournal.pmed.1001214.

Behague, D.P. and K.T. Storeng (2008). Collapsing the vertical-horizonthal divide: an ethnographic study of evidence-based policymaking in maternal health. *American Journal of Public Health* 98(4), 644–649.

Behague, D., C. Tawiah, and M. Rosato (2009). Evidence-based policy-making: the implications of globally-applicable research for context-specific problem-solving in developing countries. *Social Science & Medicine* 69, 1539–1546.

Berman, P. (1982). Selective primary health care: is efficient sufficient? *Social Science & Medicine* 16, 1054–1058.

Berman, P. and R. Ahuja (2008). Government health spending in India. *Economic and Political Weekly* 46, 26–27.

Bhattarcharya, S. (2004). Uncertain advances: a review of the final phases of the smallpox eradication program in India, 1960–1980. *American Journal of Public Health* 94(11), 1875–1883.

Bines, J. (2006). Intussusception and rotavirus vaccines. *Vaccine* 24, 3772–3776.

Birn, A.-E. (2009). The stages of international (global) health: Histories of success or successes of history? *Global Public Health* 4, 50–68.

Birn, A.-E. (2011). Small(pox) success? *Ciência & Saúde Coletiva* 16(2), 591–597.

Bisht, S. and L. Coutinho (2000). When cure is better than prevention: immunity and preventive care of measles, *Economic and Political Weekly* 35(8/9), 697–708.

Blume, S.S. (2005). Lock in, the state, and vaccine development: lessons from the history of the polio vaccines. *Research Policy* 34, 159–173.

Blume, S.S. (2006). Anti-vaccination movements and their interpretations. *Social Science & Medicine* 62, 628–642.

Blume, S.S. (2008) Toward a history of 'the vaccine innovation system', 1950–2000, in C. Hannaway (ed.), *Biomedicine in the Twentieth Century: Practices, Policies and Politics*, pp. 255–286. Amsterdam, Berlin and Oxford: IOS Press.

Blume, S.S. and J. Tump (2010). Evidence and policymaking. The introduction of MMR vaccine in the Netherlands. *Social Science & Medicine* 71, 1049–1055.

Blume, S.S. and M. Zanders (2006). Vaccine independence, local competences and globalisation. Lessons from the history of pertussis vaccine. *Social Science & Medicine* 63, 1825–1835.

Bøås, M. and D. McNeill (eds) (2004). *Global Institutions and Development: Framing the World?* London: Routledge.

Bosch-Capblanch, X., M. Kelly, and P. Garner (2011). Do existing research summaries on health systems match immunisation managers' needs in middle- and low-income countries? Analysis of 2007 health systems strengthening support. *BMC Public Health* Article Number 449, June 8 2011.

Bose, A. (2005). Private health sector in India: is private health care at the cost of public healthcare? *British Medical Journal* 331(7528), 1338–1339.

Boseley, S. (2011). *The Guardian*, June 6. Available at http://www.guardian.co.uk/society/2011/jun/06/analysis-vaccination-programmes. Accessed 6 April 2012.

Bowie, C., D.P. Mathanga, and H. Misiri (2006). Poverty, access and immunisations in Malawi—a descriptive study. *Malawi Medical Journal* 8(1), 19–27.

Brada, B. (2011). Not *here*: making the spaces and subjects of 'global health' in Botswana. *Culture, Medicine and Psychiatry* 35, 285–312.

Bresee, J.S., U.D. Parashar, and M.-A. Widdowson et al. (2005). Update on rotavirus vaccines. *Pediatric Infectious Disease Journal* 24(11), 947–952.

Brooks, A. and A. Ba-Nguz (2012). Country planning for health interventions under development: lessons from the malaria vaccine decision-making framework and implications for other new interventions. *Health Policy and Planning* 27, ii50–ii61.

Brown, L.D. (2010). The political face of public health. *Public Health Reviews* 32, 155–173.

Brown, T.M., M. Cueto, and E. Fee (2006). The World Health Organization and the transition from international to global public health. *American Journal of Public Health* 96(1), 62–72.

Brugha, R., M. Starling, and G. Walt (2002). GAVI, the first steps: lessons for the global fund. *The Lancet* 359, 435–438.

Bryson, M., P. Duclos, and A. Jolly (2010a). Global immunization policy making processes. *Health Policy* 96, 154–159.

Bryson, M., P. Duclos, A. Jolly, and N. Cakmak (2010b). A global look at the national Immunization Technical Advisory Groups. *Vaccine* 285, A13–A17.

Bull, B. and D. McNeill (2007). *Development Issues in Global Governance: Market Multilateralism and Public-Private Partnerships*. London: Routledge.

Burchett, H.E.D., S. Mounier-Jack, U.K. Griffiths, and A.J. Mills (2012a). National decision-making on adopting new vaccines: a systematic review. *Health Policy and Planning* 27, ii62–ii76.

Burchett, H.E.D. et al. (2012b). New vaccine adoption: qualitative study of national decision-making processes in seven low-and middle-income countries. *Health Policy and Planning* 27, ii5–ii16.

Buse, K. and Walt, G. (2000). Global public-private partnerships: part 1—a new development in health? *Bulletin of the World Health Organization* 78, 549–561.

Byskov J., A. Bloch, and A. Blystad et al. (2009). Accountability setting for trust in health systems-the need for research into a new approach for strengthening sustainability health action in developing countries. *Health Research Policy and Systems* 7(23), Available at http://www.health-policy-systems.com/content/pdf/1478-4505-7-23.pdf.

Caines, K. and N'jie, H. (2002). *Report of the External Review of the Functions and Interactions of the GAVI Working Group, Secretariat and Board*. GAVI.

Calain, P. (2006a). Exploring the international arena of global public health surveillance. *Health Policy and Planning* 22, 2–12.

Calain, P. (2006b). From the field side of the binoculars: a different view on global public health surveillance. *Health Policy and Planning* 22, 13–20.

Cambridge Economic Policy Associates (2010). Second GAVI Evaluation. Available at http://www.gavialliance.org/resources/GAVI_Second_Evaluation_Report_Final_13Sep2010.pdf.

Carlson, C., M. Boivin, A. Chirwa et al. (2008). *Malawi Health SWAp Mid-Term Review: Summary Report*. NORAD Collected Reviews 32/2008. Oslo, Norway.

Center for Vaccine Ethics and Policy (2011). Quoting a report by a market research firm, Research & Markets. Available at http://centerforvaccineethicsandpolicy.wordpress.com. Accessed April 2012.

Chataway, J., R. Hanlin, J. Mugwagwa, and L. Muraguri (2010). Global health social technologies: reflections on evolving theories and landscapes. *Research Policy* 39, 1277–1288.

Chatterjee, P. (2004). Delhi Lecture. Available at http://www.globalcult.org.ve/doc/Partha/Partha_1.pdf. Accessed 3 April 2012.

Chee, G., N. His, K. Carlson, S. Chankova, and P. Taylor (2008). *Evaluation of the GAVI Phase 1 Performance (2000—2005)*. Cambridge MA: Abt Associates.

Chilowa, W. and A. Munthali (1998). *A study of vaccination cultures, social demand for immunization and practices of vaccination regimes: Ntchisi district report*. Zomba: Centre for Social Research.

Chittangia, R. (2009) *Delhi steps up vigil against swine flu*. In: *Times of India Delhi* June 13. Avaiable at http://articles.timesofindia.indiatimes.com/2009-06-13/delhi/28157371_1_thermal-scanners-swine-flu-vineet-choudhary.

Clemens, M., C.H. Kenny, and T.J. Moss (2007). The trouble with the MDGs: confronting expectations of aid and development success. *World Development* 35(5), 735–751.

Corbridge, S., G. Williams, M. Srivastava, and R. Veron (2005). *Seeing the State: Governance and Governmentality in India*. Cambridge: Cambridge University Press.

Coutinho, L., S. Bisht, and G. Raje (2000). Numerical narratives and documentary practices: vaccines, targets and reports on immunization coverage. *Economic and Political Weekly* 35(8, 9), 656–666.

Cox, R.W. (ed.) (1997). *The New Realism: Perspectives on Multilateralism and World Order*. New York: Macmillan and United Nations University Press.

Cueto, M. (2004). The origins of primary health care and selective primary health care. *American Journal of Public Health* 94, 1864–1874.

Cunliffe, N. and O. Nakagomi (2007). Introduction of rotavirus vaccines in developing countries: remaining challenges. *Annals of Tropical Paediatrics* 27, 157–167.

Daily Times (2007). Available at http://groups.yahoo.com/group/MALAWIANA/message/17889. Accessed 23 July 2012.

Danielsen, L. (2011). *Children of Satan, Mothers of the Barren Land: An Analysis of Women and Child Witchcraft in a Malawian Village*. Master's Thesis, Department of Social Anthropology, University of Oslo. Oslo: University of Oslo, p. 111.

Das, J. and S. Das (2003) Trust, learning and vaccination: Evidence from a North Indian Village. *Social Science and Medicine* 57, 97–112.

Das, V. (1989). *What Do We Mean by Health?* Canberra: Australian National University.

Das, R.K. and P. Dasgupta (2000). Child health and immunisation. A macro-perspective. *Economic and Political Weekly* 35(8–9), 645–655.

Das,V., R.K. Das, and L. Coutinho (2000). Disease control and immunization, a sociological inquiry. *Economic and Political Weekly* 35(8–9), 625–632.

das Gupta, M. (2005). *Public Health in India: An Overview*. World Bank Policy Research Working Paper No. 3787. Washington DC: World Bank (Development Research Group).

Davey Smith, G., A. Gorter., J. Hoppenbrouwer et al. (1993). The cultural construction of childhood diarrhoea in rural Nicaragua: relevance for epidemiology and health promotion. *Social Science & Medicine* 36(12), 1613–1624.

de Oliviera, L.H., M.C. Danovaro-Holliday, N.J. Sanwogou et al. (2011). Progress in the introduction of rotavirus vaccine in Latin America and the Caribbean. *Pediatric Infectious Disease Journal* (Supplement) 30(1), S61–S66.

Devraj, R. (2012). *India serves up costly cocktail of vaccines*. Rome: Inter Press Service, April 27.

DLHS-3 (2007–2008). District level household and facility survey. Available at www.rchiips. org. Accessed on 15 March 2012.

Druce, N., C. Atim, C. Grace, T.J. Olsen, E. Karim, G., Murindwa, M. Sakho, and C. Sambo (2006). *Evidence-informed decision-making processes for new vaccines and other technologies:Strengthening capacity at country level*. Synthesis report. London: HLSP.

Durbach, N. (2000). They might as well brand us. Working class resistance to compulsory vaccination in Victorian England. *Social History of Medicine* 13, 45–62.

Eggen, Ø. (2011). *Dissonance in Development: Foreign Aid and State Formation in Malawi*. Ås: Norwegian University of Life Sciences.

Eie, E. (2008). *Vaccine Introduction at Country Level; A Case Study in Malawi*. Department of General Practice and Community Medicine, Section for International Health. Oslo, Norway, University of Oslo, Faculty of Medicine. Master of Philosophy: 118

Englund, H. (2006). *Prisoners of Freedom: Human Rights and the African Poor*. Berkeley, CA: University of California Press.

Erasmus, E. and L. Gilson (2008). How to start thinking about investigating power in the organizational settings of policy implementation *Health Policy and Planning* 23, 361–368.

Esser, D.E. and K.K. Bench (2011). Does global health funding respond to recipients' needs? Comparing public and private donor's allocations in 2005–2007 *World Development* 39(8), 1271–1280.

Fairhead, H.M. and M. Small (2004). Childhood Vaccination and Society in the Gambia: Public Engagement with Science and Delivery. *IDS Working Paper* 218, Brighton: UK.

Feachem, R. and O. Sabot (2006). An examination of the Global Fund at 5 years. *The Lancet* 368(9534), 537–540.

Fenner, F. (1996). Smallpox eradication: the vindication of Jenner's prophecy, in S.A. Plotkin and B. Fantini (eds), *Vaccinia, Vaccination, Vaccinology. Jenner, Pasteur and their successors*, pp. 73–78. Amsterdam: Elsevier.

Ferguson, J. and A. Gupta (2002). Spatializing states: Towards an ethnography of neo-liberal governmentality. *American Ethnologist* 29(4), 981–1002.

Fidler, D.P. (2004). *SARS, Governance and the Globalization of Disease*. London: Palgrave Macmillan.

Fidler, D.P. (2011). Rise and fall of global health as a foreign policy issue. *Global Health Governance* IV(2). Available at http://ghgj.org/DavidFidler.pdf.

Fidler, D.P. and L.O. Gostin (2006). The new International Health Regulations: An historic development for international law and public health. *Journal of Law, Medicine & Ethics* 34, 85–94.

Foege, W. (1985). Applied research, in Task Force for Child Survival. *Protecting the World's Children*, p. 167. Cartagena: Bellagio II.

Foege, W.H., J.D. Millar, and D.A. Henderson (1975). Smallpox eradication in West and Central Africa. *Bulletin of the World Health Organization* 52, 209–222.

Galazka, A., J. Milstein, and M. Zaffran (2006). *Temperature sensitivity of vaccines. Global Programme for Vaccines and Immunisation.* Geneva: World Health Organisation.

Gauri, V. and P. Khaleghian (2002). Immunization in developing countries: its political and organizational determinants. *World Development* 30(12), 2109–2132.

GAVI (2005). *17th GAVI Board Meeting and Joint Alliance Fund Board Meeting Report, 6–7 December, New Delhi, India.* Geneva: GAVI Alliance.

GAVI (2010). *Alliance Annual Financial Report.* Available at http://www.gavialliance.org/funding/financial-reports/.

GAVI Alliance (2009). *18 million Indian children to receive life-saving five-in-one vaccine.* Geneva. The Gavi Alliance: Geneva. Available at www.gavialliance.org. Accessed 10 February 2011.

GAVI Alliance (2012). *India Strategy Update. Report to the GAVI Alliance Board. 12-13 June 2012.* Available at www.gavialliance.org. Accessed August 2012.

George, A. (2009). 'By papers and pens, you can do only so much': Views about accountability and human resource management from Indian Government health administration and workers. *International Journal of Health Planning and Management* 24, 205–224.

Gessner, B.D., Duclos, P., DeRoeck, D., and Nelson, A. (2010). Informing decision makers: Experience and process of 15 National Immunization Technical Advisory Groups. *Vaccine* 285, A1–A5.

Gezondheidsraad (2007). *De toekomst van het Rijksvaccinatieprogramma: Naar een programma voor alle leeftijden.* [The future of the national vaccination programme: Towards a programme for all age groups]. The Hague: Health Council.

Ghosh, I. and L. Coutinho (2000). Normalcy and crisis in time of Cholera. An ethnography of Cholera in Calcutta. *Economic and Political Weekly* 35(8–9), 684–696.

Gish, O. (1982). Selective primary health care: old wine in new bottles. *Social Science & Medicine* 16, 1049–1063.

Gjostein, D. (2012). *Negotiating conflicting roles: Female community health workers in rural Rajasthan. A perspective on the Indian ASHA-programme.* Department of Social Anthropology, Oslo, Norway, University of Oslo. Master, 2012.

Gjostein, D., S. Knivestøen, and C. Nordfeldt (2010). *India: Local vaccination interfaces: Vaccination day in a Rajasthani village.* Working paper, Sum Medic Annual Workshop, New Delhi, 17–18/2/2011.

Glass, R., J.S. Bresee, and R. Turcios et al. (2005). Rotavirus vaccines: targeting the developing world. *Journal of Infectious Diseases* 192(Supplement 1), S160–S166.

Global Economic Governance (2008). *Setting a Developing Country Agenda for Global Health: Preliminary Report of a High-Level Working Group,* 11–13 May 2008. Global Economic Governance Programme of Oxford University Oxford.

Gloyd, S., T. Suarez, J. Torres, and M.A. Mercer (2003). Immunization campaigns and political agendas: Retrospective from Ecuador and El Salvador. *International Journal of Health Services* 33, 113–128.

Goetz, A.M. and R. Jenkins (2011). Hybrid forms of accountability: citizen engagement in institutions of public-sector oversight in India. *Public Management Review* (3)3, 363–383.

Goldman, M. (2005). *Imperial Nature. The World Bank and Struggles for Social Justice in the Age of Globalization.* New Haven: Yale University Press.

Government of India (1946). *Report of the Health Survey and Development Committee, Vol II*. New Delhi: Manager of Publications.

Government of India (1988). *National Mission on Immunization*. MoHFW, New Delhi.

Government of India (2008). *Social Sector. Planning Commission, Vol. 2*. Eleventh five-year plan, 2007–2012, pp. 57–107. New Delhi: Oxford University Press.

Gradmann, C. and V. Hess (eds) (2008). Vaccines as medical, industrial, and administrative objects. *Science in Context* (Special issue) 21, 2.

Greenough, P. (1995a). Intimidation, coercion and resistance in the final stages of the South Asian smallpox eradication campaign, 1973–1975. *Social Science & Medicine* 41(5), 633–645.

Greenough, P. (1995b). Global immunization and culture: compliance and resistance in large scale public health campaigns. *Social Science & Medicine* 41(5), 605–607.

Grundy, J. (2010). Country-level governance of global health initiatives: an evaluation of immunization coordination mechanisms in five countries of Asia. *Health Policy and Planning* 25, 185–196.

Gupta, A. (1995). Blurred boundaries: the discourse of corruption, the culture of politics, and the imagined state. *American Ethnologist* 22, 375–402.

Gupta, M. (2002). *State health systems: Orissa*, Working Paper No. 89. New Delhi: Indian Council for Research on International Economic Relations.

Gupta, D.M., V. Ramachandran, and R.K. Muthatar (2001). Epidemiological Profile of India: Historical and Contemporary Perspectives. *Journal of Biosciences* 26(4), 437–464.

Haas, E.B. (1990). *When Knowledge Is Power: Three Models of Change in International Organizations*. Berkeley: University of California Press.

Haas, P. (1992). Epistemic communities and international policy coordination. *International Organization* 46(1), 1–35.

Haas, P. (ed.) (1997). *Knowledge, Power, and International Policy Coordination*. Columbia: University of South Carolina Press.

Haas, M., T. Ashton, and K. Blum et al. (2009). Drugs, sex, money and power: an HPV vaccine case study. *Health Policy* 92, 288–295.

Hardon, A.P. and S.S. Blume (2005). Shifts in global immunization goals (1984–2004): unfinished agendas and mixed results. *Social Science & Medicine* 60, 345–356.

Henderson, R.H. (1984). The Expanded Program on Immunization of the World Health Organization. *Reviews of Infectious Diseases* 6(Supplement 2), S475–S479.

Hermann, K., W. Van Damme, G.W. Pariyo, E. Schouten, Y. Assefa, A. Cicera, and W. Massavon (2009). Community health workers for ART in sub-Saharan Africa: learning from experience—capitalizing on new opportunities. *Human Resources for Health* 7(31). doi:10.1186/1478-4491-7-31.

Hill, P.S. (2002). The rhetoric of sector-wide approaches for health development. *Social Science & Medicine* 54, 1725–1737.

Hinman, A.R., W.H. Foege, C.A. De Quadros, et al. (1987). The case for global eradication of poliomyelitis. *Bulletin of the World Health Organization* 65, 835–840.

HLSP (2005). *Lessons Learned from GAVI Phase 1 and Design of Phase 2: Findings from the Country Consultation Process*. Report to GAVI Secretariat. London: HLSP.

Horton, R. and P. Das (2011a). The Vaccine Paradox. *The Lancet* 378, 296–298.

Horton, R. and P. Das (2011b). Indian health: the path from crisis to progress. *The Lancet* 377(9761), 181–183.

Hutton, G. and M. Tanner (2004). The sector-wide approach: a blessing for public health? *Bulletin of the World Health Organization* 82, 12.

Inda, J.X. and R. Rosaldo (2008). Tracking global flows, in J.X. Inda and R. Rosaldo (eds), *The Anthropology of Globalization. A Reader*, pp. 3–46. Oxford: Blackwell Publishing.

International Institute for Population Sciences (IIPS) and Macro International (2007). *National Family Health Survey (NFHS-3), 2005–06, India: Key Findings.* Mumbai: IIPS.

Jackson, J.T. (2005). *The Globalizers: Development Workers in Action.* Baltimore: Johns Hopkins University Press.

Jain, S.K. et al. (2006). Child survival and safe motherhood program in Rajasthan. *Indian Journal of Paediatrics* 73, 43–48.

James F., M. Leach and M. Small (2004). *Childhood vaccination and society in The Gambia: public engagement with science and delivery,* IDS working paper 218. Brighton, UK: University of Sussex.

Jamison, D.T., J. Frenk, and F. Knaul (1998). International collective action in health: objectives, functions and rationale. *The Lancet* 351, 514–517.

Jeppsson, A., H. Birungi, P.-O. Östergren, and B. Hagström (2005). The global-local dilemma of a Ministry of Health: Experience from Uganda. *Health Policy* 72, 311–320.

John, J.T. (2010). India's National Technical Advisory Group on Immunization. *Vaccine* 28(Supplement 1), A88–A90.

Justice, J. (2000a). The politics of child survival, in L.M. Whiteford and L. Manderson (eds), *Global Policy/Local Realities: The Fallacy of the Level Playing Field.* Boulder, CO: Lynne Rienner Press.

Justice, J. (2000b). *Summary of the Studies of Factors Influencing the Introduction of New and Underutilized Vaccines.* Study Commissioned by Children's Vaccine Initiative and USAID's Children's Vaccine Program. Geneva: Children's Vaccine Initiative.

Kadzandira, J.M and W.R. Chilowa (2001). *The role of Health Surveillance Assistants (HSAs) in the delivery of health services and immunization in Malawi,* p. 84. Lilongwe: Centre for Social Research.

Kaler, A. (2009). Health interventions and the persistence of rumour. The circulation of sterility stories in African public health. *Social Science & Medicine* (Special issue) 68, 1711–1719.

Katsulukuta, A. (2011). *Malawi: Making use of community health workers to improve coverage— opportunities and challenges,* presentation at the The Global Immunization Meeting. 1-3 February. Geneva: WHO available at. http://www.who.int/immunization_delivery/ systems_policy/Making_use_community_health_Malawi.pdf (accessed on Apil 18 2012)

Kauchali, S., N. Rollins, and J. Van den Broeck (2004). Local beliefs about childhood diarrhoea: importance for healthcare and research. *Journal of Tropical Pediatrics* 50(2), 82–89.

Kaul, I. (2006). Blending domestic and external policy demands: The rise of the intermediary state, in I. Kaul and P. Conceicao (eds), *The New Public Finance: Responding to Global Challenges.* New York: Oxford University Press.

Keugoung, B., J. Macq, A. Bove, J. Meli, and C. Bart (2011). The interface between health systems and vertical programmes in Francophone Africa: the managers' perceptions. *Tropical Medicine and International Health* 16(4), 476–485.

Kickbusch, I., W. Hein, and G. Silberschmidt (2010). Addressing global health governance challenges through a new mechanism: The proposal for a Committee C of the World Health Assembly. *Journal of Law Medicine & Ethics* 38(3), 550–563.

Knivstøen, S. (2012). *Pregnancy, Delivery & Family Planning: A study of health seeking behaviour in Meopur village in Rajasthan, India*. Department of Social Anthropology, Oslo, Norway (unpublished thesis), University of Oslo, Master.

Koplan, J.P., T.C. Bond, M.H. Merson, et al. (2009). Towards a common definition of global health. *Lancet* 373 (9679), 1993–1995.

Labontè, R. (2008). Global health in public policy. Finding the right frame? *Critical Public Health* 18(4), 467–482.

Labonté, R. and M. Gagnon (2010). Framing health and foreign policy: lessons for global health diplomacy. *Globalization and Health* 6, 14.

Lahariya, C. (2007). Global eradication of polio: the case for 'finishing the job'. *Bulletin of the World Health Organization* 85(6), 487–492.

Lakoff, A. (2010). Two regimes of global health. *Humanity: An international Journal of Human Rights, Humanitarianism and Development* 1(1), 59–79.

Langsten, R. and K. Hill (1995). Treatment of childhood diarrhea in rural Egypt. *Social Science & Medicine* 40, 989–1001.

Leach, M. and J. Fairhead (2005). *The cultural and political dynamics of technology delivery: The case of infant immunization in Africa*. Project funded by the Committee on Social Science Research, DFID, Research Report. Brighton, UK: IDS, University of Sussex.

Leach, M. and J. Fairhead (2007). *Vaccine Anxieties. Global Science, Child Health and Society*. London: Earthscan.

Lele, U., R. Ridker, and J. Upadhyay (2005). Health system capacities in developing countries and global health initiatives on communicable diseases. Background paper prepared for the International Task Force on Public Goods. Available at http://www.umalele.org/publications/health_system_capacities.pdf.

Lim, S., D. Stein, A. Charrow, and C. Murray (2008). Tracking progress towards universal childhood immunisation and the impact of global initiatives: a systematic analysis of three-dose diphtheria, tetanus, and pertussis immunisation coverage. *The Lancet* 372(9655), 2031–2046.

Lob-Levyt, J. (2009) Vaccine coverage and the GAVI Alliance Immunization Services Support Initiative. *The Lancet*, 373(9659), 209.

Lone, Z. and J.M Puliyel (2010). Introducing pentavalent vaccine in the EPI in India: A counsel for caution. *Indian Journal of Medical Research*

Long, N. (1989) *Encounters at the Interface: A perspective on Social Discontinuities in Rural development*. Wageningen Studies in Sociology no.27. Wageningen: Wageningen Agricultural University.

Long, N. (2001). *Development Sociology: Actors Perspectives*. London: Routledge

Long, N. (2004). Contesting policy ideas from below, in M. Bøås and D. McNeill (eds), *Global Institutions and Development*. London: Routledge.

Lwanda, J. (2007). Scotland, Malawi and medicine: Livingston's legacy, I presume? An historical perspective. *Scottish Medical Journal* 52(3), 36–44.

Lydon, P., R. Levine, M. Makinen, et al. (2008). Introducing new vaccines in the poorest countries: What did we learn from the GAVI experience with financial sustainability? *Vaccine* 26, 6706–6716.

Madhavi, Y. (2003). Manufacture of consent? Hepatitis B vaccination. *Economic & Political Weekly* 14 June, 2417–2424.

Madhavi, Y. (2005). Vaccine Policy in India. *PloS Medicine* 2(5), e127. doi:10.1371/journal.pmed.0020127.

Madhavi, Y. and N. Raghuram (2010). Pentavalent and other new combination vaccines. Solutions in search of problems. *Indian Journal of Medical Research* 132, 456–457.

Madhavi, Y., J. Puliyel, J.L. Mathew, N. Raghuram (2010). Evidence-based national vaccine policy. *Indian Journal of Medical Research* 131, 617–628.

Mahler, H. (2008). Former WHO director Halfdan Mahler on Alma Ata, May 2008. http://www.socialmedicine.org/2008/06/11/globalization-and-health/former-who-director-halfdan-mahler-on-alma-ata-phc-may-2008. Accessed April 2012.

Mahoney, R. (2004). Policy analysis: An essential research tool for the introduction of vaccines in developing countries. *Journal of Health, Population and Nutrition* 22, 331–337.

Makinen, M., M. Kaddar, V. Molldrem, and L. Wilson (2012). New vaccine adoption in lower-middle-income countries. *Health Policy and Planning* 27, ii39–ii49.

Malawi Ministry of Health (2004a). *A Joint Program of Work for a health sector-wide approach (SWAp) 2004–2010*. Department of Planning, Ministry of Health, Lilongwe, Malawi.

Malawi Ministry of Health (2004b). *Financial Sustainability Plan (FSP) for Expanded Programme of Immunization (EPI)*. Malawi.

Malawi Multiple Indicator Cluster Survey (2004). *Monitoring the situation of Children and women*. Zomba: NSO.

Malawi National Statistical Office (2005). *Malawi Demographic and Health Survey 2004*. Calverton, MD: NSO and ORC Marco.

Malawi National Statistical Office (2011). *Malawi Population and Housing Census 2008*. Integrated Public Use Microdata Series, International: Version 6.1. Minneapolis: Minnesota Population Center, University of Minnesota.

Malawi National Statistical Office (2011). *Malawi Demographic and Health Survey 2010*. Calverton, MD: NSO and ORC Macro.

Malik, G. (2009). The role of auxiliary nurse midwives in national rural health mission. *Nursing Journal of India* C(3). http://www.tnaionline.org/april-09/8.htm. Accessed 15 July 2010.

Mansoor, O., S. Shin, C. Maher (2000). *Asessing new vaccines for national immunisation programmes: A framework to assist decision-makers*. Manila: WHO Regional Office for the Western Pacific.

Marchel, B., K. Cavalli, and G. Kegels (2009). Global health actors claim to support health system strengthening—is this reality or rhetoric? *PLoS Medicine* 6(4), e1000059. doi:10.371/journal.pmed.1000059.

Markowitz, L. E., J. Sepulveda, et al. (1990). Immunization of six-month-old infants with different doses of Edmonston-Zagreb and Schwarz measles vaccines. *New England Journal of Medicine* 322(9), 580–587.

McCoy, D., S. Chand, and D. Sridhar (2009). Global health funding: how much, where it comes from and where it goes. *Health Policy and Planning* 24, 407–417.

McKinsey and Company (2003). *Achieving our Immunization Goal: Final Report*. Washington DC: McKinsey and Company.

McMichael, A.J. (2000). The urban environment and health in a world of increasing globalization: issues for developing countries. *Bulletin of the World Health Organization* 78, 1117–1123.

McNeill, D. (1981). *The Contradictions of Foreign Aid*. London: Croom Helm.

McNeill, D. and A. L. St Clair (2009). *Global Poverty, Ethics and Human Rights: The Role of Multilateral Organisations*. London: Routledge.

McVea, K.L.S.P. (1997). Lay injection practices among migrant farm workers in the age of AIDS: Evolution of a biomedical folk practice. *Social Science & Medicine* 45(1), 91–98.

Mills, A. (1983). Vertical vs horizonthal health programmes in Africa: Idealism, pragmatism, resources,and efficiency. *Social Science & Medicine* 17(24), 1971–1981.

Mills, A., F. Rasheed, and S. Tollman (2007). *Strengthening Health Systems. Disease Control Priorities in Developing Countries*, 2nd edition. Available at http://www.dcp2.org/pubs/DCP.

Milstien, J.B., L. Kamara, P. Lydon, V. Mitchell, and S. Landry (2008). The GAVI Financing Task Force: One model of partner collaboration. *Vaccine* 26, 5296–5302.

Mishra, A. (2010). *Hunger and famine in Kalahandi: An anthropological study*. New Delhi: Pearson Longman.

Mishra, A. and S. Sarma (2011). Understanding health and illness among tribal communities in Orissa. *Indian Anthropologist* 41(2), 1–16.

MoH (2002). *Republic of Malawi Ministry of Health and Population, Expanded Programme on Immunization*, Malawi Field Operational Manual, Lilongwe, Malawi.

MoH (2003). *Malawi National Immunisation Programme: Financial Sustainability Plan*. Lilongwe, Malawi. http://www.who.int/immunization_financing/countries/mwi/malawi_fsp.pdf.

MoH (2004). *A Joint Programme of Work for a health sector-wide approach (SWAp) 2004–2010*. Department of Planning, Ministry of Health, Lilongwe, Malawi.

MoH (2010). *Dowa District EPI Performance Annual Review 2010*. Lilongwe, Malawi.

MoHFW (2002–03), Annual Report (2002–03), Ministry of Health and Family Welfare, Government of India.

MoHFW (2005–06). *Annual Report (2005–06)*, Ministry of Health and Family Welfare, Government of India.

MoHFW (2006). *Child Health in Government of India 2006 Family Welfare Statistics*, Chapter 9. Available at http://hetv.org/india/nfhs/nfhs3/NFHS-3-Chapter-09-Child-Health.pdf.

MoHFW (2011). *National Vaccine Policy*. Government of India.

Moser, K.A., D.A. Leon, and D.R. Gwatkin (2005). How does progress toward the child mortality millennium development goal affect inequalities between the poorest and the least poor? Analysis of demographic and health survey data. *British Medical Journal* 331, 1180–1182.

Moulin, A.-M. (2004). The international network of the Pasteur Institute, scientific innovations and French tropisms, in C. Charle, J. Schriewer, and P. Wagner (eds), *The Emergence of Transnational Intellectual Networks and the Cultural Logic of Nations*, pp. 135–162. New York: Campus Verlag.

Mudur, G. (2010). Antivaccine lobby resists introduction of Hib-vaccine in India. *British Medical Journal* 340, c3508.

Munira, S.L. and S.A. Fritzen (2007). What influences government adoption of vaccines in developing countries? A policy process analysis. *Social Science & Medicine* 65, 1751–1764.

Munthali, A. (2007). Determinants of Vaccination Coverage in Malawi: Evidence from the Demographic and Health Surveys. *Malawi Medical Journal* 19(2), 79–82.

Munthali, S. and B. Johns (2011). *The Cost of Child Health Services in Four Districts of Malawi: Baseline data for Estimating the Cost and Cost-effectiveness of the Rapid Scale-up for Child Health*. Final Report July 2011. Department of Economics, Zomba Chancellor College, University of Malawi (unpublished).

Muraskin, W. (1998). *The Politics of International Health: the Children's Vaccine Initiative and the Struggle to Develop Vaccines for the Third World*. Albany: State University of New York Press.

Muraskin, W. (2002) in M. Reich (ed.), *The Last Years of the CVI and the Birth of the GAVI. Public-Private Partnerships for Public Health*, Chapter 6. pp. 115–168. Cambridge, MA: Harvard Centre for Population Studies.

Muraskin, W. (2004). The global alliance for vaccines and immunization: Is it a new model for effective public-private cooperation in international public health? *American Journal of Public* Health 94(11), 1922–1925.

Muraskin, W. (2005). *Crusade to Immunize the World's Children: the Origin of the Bill and Melinda Gates Children's Vaccine Program and the Birth of the Global Alliance for Vaccines and Immunization*. Los Angeles: University of Southern California, Marshall School, Global BioBusinessbook.

Muraskin, W. (2012). *Polio Eradication and its Discontents*. New Delhi: Orient BlackSwan.

Naimoli, J.F. (2009). Global health partnerships in practice: taking stock of the GAVI Alliance's new investment in health systems strengthening. *International Journal of Health Planning and Management* 24(1), 3–25.

Nair, H., I. Hazarika, and A. Patwari (2011). A roller-coaster ride: Introduction of pentavalent vaccine in India. *Journal of Global Health* 1, 32–35.

National Statistical Office (Malawi), Minnesota Population Center (2011). *Malawi Population and Housing Census 2008*. Integrated Public Use Microdata Series, International: Version 6.1 Minneapolis: University of Minnesota.

Newell, K.W. (1988). Selective primary health care: the counter revolution. *Social Science & Medicine* 26, 903–906.

Nichter, M. (1990). Vaccinations in South Asia: False expectations and commanding metaphors, in J. Coreil and J. Dennis Mull (eds), *Anthropology and Primary Health Care*, pp. 196–221. Boulder: Westview Press.

Nichter, M. (1995). Vaccinations in the third world: a consideration of community demand. *Social Science & Medicine* 41, 617–632.

Nordfeldt, C. and S. Roalkvam (2010). Choosing vaccination: Negotiating child protection and good citizenship in modern India. *Forum for Development Studies* 37(3), 327–347.

Nyirenda, L. and R. Flikke (2012). Frontline vaccinators and Immunisation Coverage in Malawi. *Forum for Development* Studies 1-20. Published online 2 October 2012. Available at http://www.tandfonline.com/doi/pdf/10.1080/08039410.2012.725676.

Nyirenda, L. and J. Justice (2012). New vaccine introduction in countries with weak health systems: the role of global health actors in Malawi. Working paper.

Obadare, E. (2005). A crisis of trust: history, politics, religion and the polio controversy in Northern Nigeria. *Patterns of Prejudice* 39, 265–284.

Okuonzi, S.A. and J. Macrae (1995). Whose policy is it anyway? International and national influences on health policy development in Uganda. *Health Policy and Planning* 10, 122–132.

Oliveira-Cruz, V., C. Kurowski, and A. Mills (2003). Delivery of priority health services: searching for synergies within the vertical versus horizontal debate. *Journal of International Development* 15, 67–86.

Ommundsen, M. (2011). *A foot in Each Camp: Health Surveillance Assistants as mediators in the social interface of child health in Malawi*. Master's thesis, Department of Social Anthropology, University of Bergen, Bergen, Norway.

Ong, A. (2007). *Neoliberalism as Exception: Mutations in Citizenship and Sovereignty*. Durham, NC: Duke University Press.

Ooms, G., W.V. Damme, B.K. Baker, P. Zeiz, and T. Schrecker (2008). The diagonal approach to Global Fund financing: a cure for the broader malaise of health systems. *Globalization and Health* 4, 6. Available at http://www.globalizationandhealth.com/content/4/1/6.

Otten, M.W., Jr., J.M. Okwo-Bele, R. Kezaala, R. Biellik, R. Eggers, and D. Nshimirimana (2003). Impact of alternative approaches accelerated measles control: experience in the African region, 1996–2002. *Journal of Infectious Disease* 187(1), S36–S43.

Otten, T. (2000). In a remote area: categories of the person and Illness among the Desia of Koraput district. *Journal of Social Sciences* 4(4), 347–356.

Otten, T. (2010). The concept of *Biba* among the Rona of Highland Orissa: wedding rituals to ensure health, in P. Berger, R. Hardenberg, E. Kattner and M. Prager (eds) *The Anthropology of Values: Essays in Honour of Georg Pfeffer*. pp 143–161. Delhi: Pearson Education.

Parashar, U.D., A. Burton, C. Lanata, et al. (2009). Global mortality associated with rotavirus disease among children in 2004. *Journal of Infectious Diseases Supplement* 1(200), S9–S15.

Paterson, P. and H.J. Larson (2012). The role of publics in the introduction of new vaccines. *Health Policy and Planning* 27, ii77–ii79.

Pathy, J. (1995). Colonial ethnography: White man's burden or political expediency. *Economic and Political Weekly* 30(4), 220–228.

Pearson, M. (2010). *DFID Impact Evaluation of the Sector Wide Approach (SWAp)*. Malawi: DFID and UKAID. Available at http://www.dfid.gov.uk/Documents/publications1/hdrc/imp-eval-sect-wde-appr-mw.pdf.

People's Health Movement (2008). *Global Health Watch 2. An Alternative World Health Report.*, Medact, Global Equity Gauge Alliance. London: Palgrave Macmillan.

Peters, D.H., A. Wagstaff, L. Pritchett, N.V. Ramana, and R.R. Sharma (2002). *Better Health Systems of India's Poor: Finding analysis and options*. New Delhi: World Bank Publication.

Pfeiffer, J. (2003). International NGOs and primary health care in Mozambique: the need for a new model of collaboration. *Social Science & Medicine* 56, 725–738.

Pickstone, J. (2011). The rule of ignorance: a polemic on medicine, English health service policy, and history. *British Medical Journal* 342, 633–634.

Program on Appropriate Technology for Health (2012). *The birth of PATH*. Available at http://www.path.org/about/birth-of-path.php. Accessed 18 October 2012.

Purohit, B. (2001). Private initiatives and policy options: recent health system experience in India. *Health Policy and Planning* 16(1), 87–97.

Quader, T. (2000). Health care systems in transition III India part I. The Indian experience. *Journal of Public Health Medicine* 22, 25–32.

Ranger, T.O. (1992). Godly medicine: the ambiguities of medical mission in southeastern Tanzania 1900–1945, in S. Feierman and J.M. Janzen (eds), *The Social Basis of Health and Healing in Africa*, pp. 256–284. Berkeley and Oxford: University of California Press.

Rao, M., A.K. Shiva Kumar, M. Chatterjee, and T. Sundararaman (2011). Human resources for health in India. *The Lancet* 377(9765), 587–598.

Ravishankar, N., P. Gubbins, R. Cooley, et al. (2009). Financing of global health: tracking development assistance for health from 1990 to 2007. *The Lancet* 373(9681), 2113–2124.

Reeler, A.V. (2000). Anthropological perspectives on injections: A review. *Bulletin of the World Health Organization* 78(1), 135–143.

Richardson, F., M. Chirwa, M. Fahnestock, M. Bishop, P. Emmart, and B. McHenry (2009). *Community-based Distribution of Injectable Contraceptives in Malawi*. Health Policy Initiative, Task Order 1. Washington, DC: Futures Group International.

Rifkin, S.B. and G. Walt (1986). Why health progress: defining the issue concerning 'Comprehensive Primary Care'. *Social Science & Medicine* 23(6), 554–566.

Roalkvam, S. (2012). Stripped of rights in the pursuit of the good: The politics of gender and the reproductive body in Rajasthan, India, in K. Bjørkdahl and K. Nilsen (eds), *Development and the Environment. Practices, Theories, Polices*, pp. 243–259. Oslo: Akademika Publishing.

Roalkvam S. and K.I. Sandberg (2010). Vaccines and the global system/or why study vaccines. *Forum for Development Studies* 37(3), 293–299.

Rosenberg, C.E. (1992). What is an epidemic? AIDS in historical perspective, in C.E. Rosenberg (ed.), *Explaining Epidemics and Other Studies in the History of Medicine*, pp. 278–292. Cambridge: Cambridge University Press.

Ruggie, J.G. (1998). *Constructing the World Polity: Essays on International Institutionalization*. London and New York: Routledge.

Ruggie, J.G. (2004). Reconstituting the global public domain—issues, actors and practices. *European Journal of International Relations* 10, 499–531.

Rugha, R., M. Starling, and G. Walt (2002). GAVI, the first steps: lessons for the Global Fund. *The Lancet* 359, 435–438.

Rushton, S. (2011). Global health security: security for whom: Security from what? *Political Studies* 59, 779–796.

Sachs, J. (2001). *Macroeconomics and Health: Investing in Health for Economic Development*. Geneva: WHO.

Samuelsen, H. (2001). Infusions of health: the popularity of vaccinations among Bissa in Burkina Faso. *Anthropology and Medicine* 8(2), 163–175.

Sandberg, K., S. Andresen, and G. Bjune (2010). A new approach to global health institutions? A case study of new vaccine introduction and the formation of the GAVI Alliance. *Social Science & Medicine* 71(7), 1349–1356.

Sarojini, N.B., S. Srinivasan, Y. Madhavi, et al. (2010). The HPV vaccine: science, ethics and regulation. *Economic & Political Weekly* 45(48), 27–34.

Sathyamala, C., O. Mittal, R. Dasgupta, and R. Priya (2005). Polio eradication initiative in India: deconstructing the GPEI. *International Journal of Health Services* 35, 361–383.

Scott, J.C. (1998). *Seeing Like a State. How Certain Schemes to Improve the Human Condition Have Failed*. New Haven: Yale University Press.

Scott Jordon, W., A. Jones, and J. Wecker (2012). Introducing multiple vaccines in low-and lower-middle-income countries: issues, opportunities and challenges. *Health Policy and Planning* 27, ii17–ii26.

Seljeskog, L., J. Sundby, and J. Chimango (2006). Factors influencing women's choice of place of delivery in rural Malawi—an explorative study. *African Journal of Reproductive Health* 10(3), 66–75.

Sen, A., (1999). *Development as Freedom*. New York: Alfred A. Knopf.

Sengupta, A. and V. Prasad (2011). Towards a truly universal Indian health system. *The Lancet* 377(9767), 702–703.

Senouci, K., J. Blau, B. Nyambat, P. Coumba Faye, L. Gautier, A.L. Da Silva, M.A. Favorov, J.M. Clemens, P.J. Stoeckel, and B. Gessner (2010). The Supporting Independent Immunization and Vaccine Advisory Committees (SIVAC) Initiative: A country driven, multi-partner programme to support evidence-based decision making. *Vaccine* 285, A26–A30.

Serquina-Ramiro, L., N. Kasniyah, T. Inthusoma, N. Higginbotham, D.L. Streiner, M. Nichter, and S. Freeman (2001). Measles immunization acceptance in Southeast Asia: Past patterns and future challenges. *Southeast Asian Journal of Tropical Medicine and Public Health* 32, 791–804.

Sharma, S. (2007). *Immunization coverage in India. Working Paper Series No. E/283/2007.* New Delhi: University of Delhi, Institute of Economic Growth. Available at http://www.iegindia.org/workpap/wp283.pdf.

Shaw, M. and I. Martin (2000). Community work, citizenship and democracy: remaking the connections. *Community Development Journal* (35)4, 401–413.

Shearer, J.C., M.L. Stack, M.R. Richmond, A.P. Bear, R.A. Hajjeh, and D.M. Bishai (2010). Accelerating Policy Decisions to Adopt *Haemophilus influenzae* Type b Vaccine: a global, multivariable analysis. PLoS Med 7(3): e1000249. doi:10.1371/journal.pmed.1000249.

Sheikh, K. and George, A. (eds) (2010). *Health Providers in India*. New Delhi: Routledge.

Shore, C. (2001). Nation and State in the European Union, in R. Kiss and A. Palàdi-Kovàcs (eds), *Times Places, Passages Ethnological Approaches in the New Millennium*, pp. 25–51. Plenary Papers of the 7th. SIEF Conference, Budapest; Akadémiai Kiadó.

Silver, G. (1998). International health services need and interorganizational policy. *American Journal of Public Health* 88, 728.

Singh, M.S. and A. Bharadwaj (2000). Communicating immunization. The mass media strategies. *Economic and Political Weekly* 35(8,9), 667–675.

Sivaramakrishnan, K. (2011). The return of epidemics and the politics of global-local health. *American Journal of Public Health* 101, 1032–1041.

Smith, J.C., D.E. Snider, and L.K. Pickering (2009). Immunization policy development in the United States: the role of the advisory committee on immunization practices. *Annals of Internal Medicine* 150, 45–49.

Soysal, Y. (1994). *Limits of Citizenship*. Chicago: University of Chicago Press.

Spicer, N. and A. Walsh (2012). 10 best resources on the current effects of global health initiatives on country health systems. *Health Policy and Planning* 27, 265–269.

Sridhar, D. (2009). Post Accra: is there space for country ownership in global health? *Third World Quarterly* 30(7), 1363–1377.

Sridhar, D. (2010). Seven Challenges in International Development Assistance for Health and Ways Forward. *Journal of Law, Medicine & Ethics* 38(3), 459–469.

Sridhar, D. and Gómez, E. (2011). Health Financing in Brazil, Russia and India: What role does the international community play? *Health Policy and Planning* 26(12), 12–24.

Starling, M., R. Brugha, and G. Walt (2002). *New products into old systems: The Global Alliance for Vaccines and Immunization (GAVI) from a country perspective*. London: Save the Children UK.

Stephenson, J. (2002). Will the current measles vaccines ever eradicate measles? *Expert Review of Vaccines* 1(3), 355–362.

Stern, A.M. and H. Markel (2005). The history of vaccines and immunization: Familiar patterns, new challenges. *Health Affairs* 24(3), 611–621.

Stone, D. and S. Maxwell (eds) (2005). *Global knowledge networks and international development: bridges across boundaries*. New York: Routledge.

Stoner, B.P. (1986). Understanding medical systems: traditional, modern and syncretic health care alternatives in medical pluralistic societies. *Medical Anthropology Quarterly* 17(2), 44–48.

Strategic Advisory Group of Experts (2012). *Session: Impact of introduction of new vaccines on the strengthening of immunization and health systems*. Available at http://www.who.int/immunization/sage/meetings/2012/april/presentations_background_docs/en/index1.html.

Streefland, P.H. (1995). Enhancing coverage and sustainability of vaccination programs: an explanatory framework with special reference to India. *Social Science & Medicine* 41, 647–657.

Streefland, P., Chowdhury, A.M.R., and P. Ramos-Jimenez (1999). Patterns of vaccine acceptance. *Social Science & Medicine* 49, 1705–1716.

Sumner, A. and T. Lawo (2010). *MDGs and Beyond: Pro-poor Policy in a Changing World*. EADI Policy Paper. http://www.eadi.org/fileadmin/Documents/Publications/policy_wp/EADI_Policy_Paper_March_2010.pdf.

Taylor, C.E., F. Cutts, and M.E. Taylor (1997). Ethical dilemmas in current planning for polio eradication. *American Journal of Public Health* 87, 922–925.

Troulliot, M.-R. (2001). The anthropology of the state in the age of globalization. *Current Anthropology* 42(1), 125–138.

UN (2010). *The Millennium Development Goals Report 2010*. New York: United Nations. Available at http://www.un.org/millenniumgoals/

UNDP (2011). *Malawi Country Profile: Human Development Indicators*. Available at http://hdrstats.undp.org/en/countries/profiles/MWI.html. Accessed 7 March 2012.

UNICEF (1990). *Why a World Summit for Children? A UNICEF perspective*. Available at http://www.cf-hst.net/unicef-temp/Doc-Repository/doc/doc349374.PDF.

UNICEF SOWC (2008). State of the World's Children. http://www.unicef.org/sowc08/

UNICEF (2011). *Health and Nutrition*. Available at http://www.unicef.org/malawi/health_nutrition.html. Accessed 8 March 2012.

UNICEF (2012). *The progress of nations*. Available at http://www.unicef.org/pon00/data9.htm. Accessed 28.20.2012.

UNICEF and National Rural Health Mission (2008). National Cold Chain Assessment India, July 2008. Available at http://www.unicef.org/india/National_Cold_Chain_Assessment_India_July_2008.pdf. New Delhi: NRHM.

UNICEF/WHO (1975) Report of meeting, document JC20/UNICEF-WHO/75.4. Joint Committee on Health Policy. New York: UNICEF.

UNICEF/WHO (2009). *Diarrhoea: Why children are still dying and what can be done*. New York and Geneva: UNICEF and WHO.

Vaccine Safety Datalink Group (2005). The use of a computerized database to monitor vaccine safety in Viet Nam. *Bulletin of the World Health Organization* 83(8), 604–608.

Vaillancourt, D. (2009). *Do Health Sector-Wide Approaches Achieve Results? Emerging Evidence and Lessons from Six Countries: Bangladesh, Ghana, Kyrgyz Republic, Malawi, Nepal, Tanzania*. Independent Evaluation Group (IEG) Working Paper 2009/4, Washington: World Bank.

Vandemoortele, J. (2011). The MDG story: intention denied. *Development and Change* 42, 1–21.

Varma, S. (2010). India rising, falling, stumbling, speeding. *The Times of India* 25 January. http://articles.timesofindia.indiatimes.com/2010-01-25/india/28129843_1_steel-production-poverty-line-economic-indicators.

Vaughan, E. and T. Tinker (2009). Influenza preparedness and response. *American Journal of Public Health Supplement* 2(99), 324–332.

Vaughn, M. (1991). *Curing their Ills: Colonial Power and African Illness*. Stanford: Stanford University Press.

Victoro, C.G., R.F. Black, J. Ties Borerma, and J. Bryce (2011). Measuring impact in the Millennium Development Goal era and beyond: a new approach to large-scale effectiveness evaluations. *The Lancet* 377, 85–95.

Vyse, A.J., N.J. Gay, J.M. White, et al. (2002). Evolution of surveillance of measles, mumps and rubella in England and Wales: providing the platform for evidence-based vaccination policy. *Epidemiologic Reviews* 24, 125–136.

Wailoo, K., J. Livingston, S. Epstein, and R. Aronowitz (eds) (2010). *Three Shots at Prevention. The HPV Vaccine and the Politics of Medicine's Simple Solutions*. Baltimore: Johns Hopkins University Press.

Waitzkin, H. (2003). Report on the WHO Commission on Macroeconomics and Health: a summary and a critique. *The Lancet* 361, 523–526.

Walsh, J. and Warren, K. S. (1979). Selective primary health care: an interim strategy for disease control in developing countries. *New England Journal of Medicine* 301, 967–974.

Walt, G. (2001). *The International Arena. Health Policy: an introduction to process and power*. London: Zed Books.

Wang, M. and S.A. Wang (2012). The privilege and responsibility of having choices: decision-making for new vaccines in developing countries. *Health Policy and Planning* 27, ii1–ii14.

Weijer, C. (2000). The future of research into rotavirus vaccine. *British Medical Journal* 321, 525–526.

Wheeler, C. and S. Berkley (2001). Initial lessons from public-private partnerships in drug and vaccine development. *Bulletin of the World Health Organization* 79, 728–733.

WHO (1976). Expanded programme on immunization. Report on a seminar organized by the WHO Regional Office for Africa. Brazzaville (unpublished).

WHO?UNICEF (1978). *Primary Health Care: Report on the international conference on Primary Health care Alma Ata*, USSR 6–12 September. Geneva: WHO.

WHO/UNICEF (2005). *Global Immunization Vision and Strategy 2006–2015*. Geneva and New York: WHO/UNICEF. Available at http://whqlibdoc.who.int/hq/2005/WHO_IVB_05.05.pdf.

Wisner, B. (1988). GOBI versus PHC? Some dangers of selective primary health care. *Social Science & Medicine* 26, 963–969.

Wonodi, C.B., I. Privor-Dumm, M. Aina, et al. (2012). Using social network analysis to examine the decision-making process on new vaccine introduction in Nigeria. *Health Policy and Planning* 27, ii27–ii38.

World Bank (1987). *Financing Health Services in Developing Countries. An Agenda for Reform*. Washington: World Bank.

World Bank (1993). *World Development Report: Investing in Health*. Washington: World Bank.

World Bank (2010). *Addressing the Electricity Access Gap: Background Paper for the World Bank Energy Sector Strategy*. Available at http://siteresources.worldbank.org/EXTESC/Resources/Addressing_the_Electricity_Access_Gap.pdf. Accessed 7 March 2012.

World Health Assembly (1976). 29th World Health Assembly. Resolutions. Geneva: WHO. Document A29/16.

World Health Assembly (1974). 27th World Health Assembly. Resolutions. Document WHA 27.57. Geneva: WHO.

World Health Organization (2000). *The World Health Report. Health Systems: improving performance*. Geneva.

World Health Organization (2002). Available at http://www.searo.who.int/LinkFiles/India_india.pdf. Accessed 2 June 2009.

World Health Organization (2008a). *International Health Regulations (2005)*, 2nd edition. Available at http://www.who.int/ihr.

World Health Organization (2008b). Sixty-first World Health Assembly. Document A61/10. Available at http://www.who.int/mediacentre/events/2008/wha61/en/index.html.

World Health Organization (2009a). Weekly Epidemiological Record, 84(23), 5 June, pp. 213–236. Geneva: WHO. Available at http://www.who.int/wer/2009/wer8423.pdf.

World Health Organization (2009b). *Detailed review paper on rotavirus vaccines'. presented to the SAGE group of experts, April*. Available at http://www.who.int/immunization/sage.

World Health Organization (2009c). *Country Cooperating Strategy 2008–2013: Malawi*. Available at http://www.who.int/countryfocus/cooperation_strategy/ccs_mwi_en.pdf. Accessed 22 March 2012.

World Health Organization (2009d). Rotavirus vaccines: an update. *Weekly Epidemiological Record* 84, 533–540.

World Health Organization (2009e). *Country Cooperation Strategy 2008–2013 Malawi*. Available at http://www.who.int/countryfocus/cooperation_strategy/ccs_mwi_en.pdf. Accessed 11 July 2012.

World Health Organization (2011a). *Country Cooperating Strategy at a Glance: Malawi*. Available at http://s.who.int/countryfocus/cooperation_strategy/ccsbrief_mwi_en.pdf. Accessed 22 March 2012.

World Health Organization (2011b). *Increasing Access to Vaccines through Technology Transfer and Local Production*. Geneva: WHO.

World Health Organization Constitution. Available at http://apps.who.int/gb/bd/PDF/bd47/EN/constitution-en.pdf.

World Health Organization, Maximising Positive Synergies Collaborative Group (2009). An assessment of interactions between global health initiatives and country health systems. *The Lancet* 373, 2137–2169.

Worst Measles Outbreak in Malawi: Death Toll 197. Submitted by hyperlink, "http://topnews.us/users/satish-karat" \o "View user profile." Satish Karat on 16 August 2010, http://topnews.us/content/224524-worst-measles-outbreak-malawi-death-toll-197.

Yahya, M. (2007). Polio vaccines—'No thank you!'. Barriers to polio eradication in Northern Nigeria. *African Affairs* 106, 185s204.

Zuber, P., I. El-Ziq, M. Kaddar, A. Ottosen, K. Rosenbaum, M. Shirey, L. Kamara, and P. Duclos (2011). Sustaining GAVI-supported vaccine introductions in resource-poor countries. *Vaccine* 29, 3149–3154.

Index